2

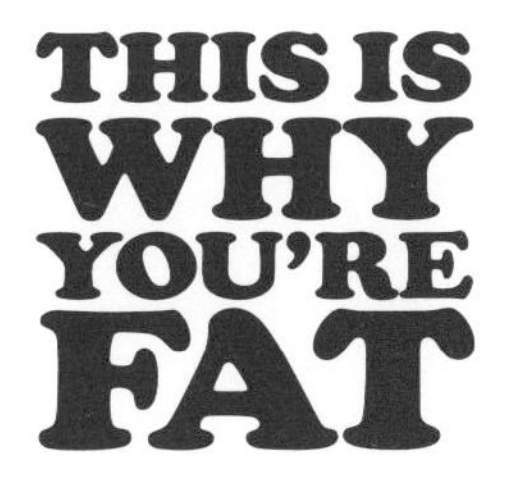

PALM BEACH COUNTY
LIBRARY SYSTEM
3650 Summit Boulevard
West Palm Beach, FL 33406-4198

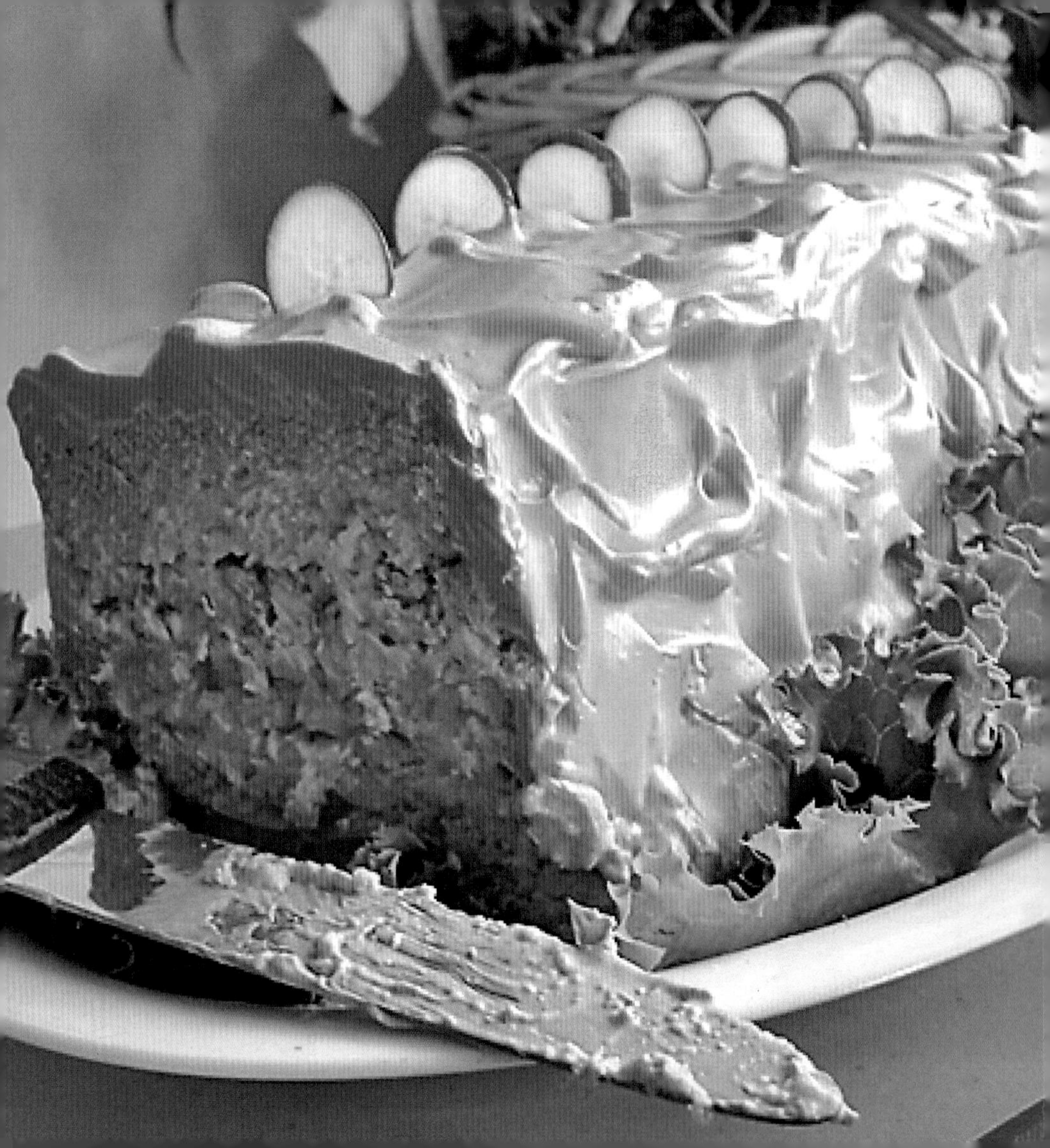

THIS IS WHY YOU'RE FAT

Where Dreams Become Heart Attacks

Jessica Amason &
Richard Blakeley

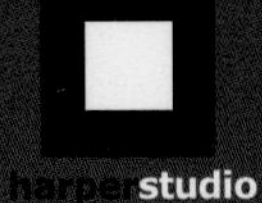

THIS IS WHY YOU'RE FAT. Copyright © 2009 by Jessica Amason and Richard Blakeley. All rights reserved. Printed in the United States of America. No part of this book may be used or reproduced in any manner whatsoever without written permission except in the case of brief quotations embodied in critical articles and reviews. For information address HarperCollins Publishers, 10 East 53rd Street, New York, NY 10022.

HarperCollins books may be purchased for educational, business, or sales promotional use. For information please write: Special Markets Department, HarperCollins Publishers, 10 East 53rd Street, New York, NY 10022.

For more information about this book or other books from HarperStudio, visit www.theharper-studio.com.

FIRST EDITION

Library of Congress Cataloging-in-Publication Data has been applied for.

ISBN 978-0-06-193663-0

09 10 11 12 13 ID/LPR 10 9 8 7 6 5 4 3 2 1

Contents

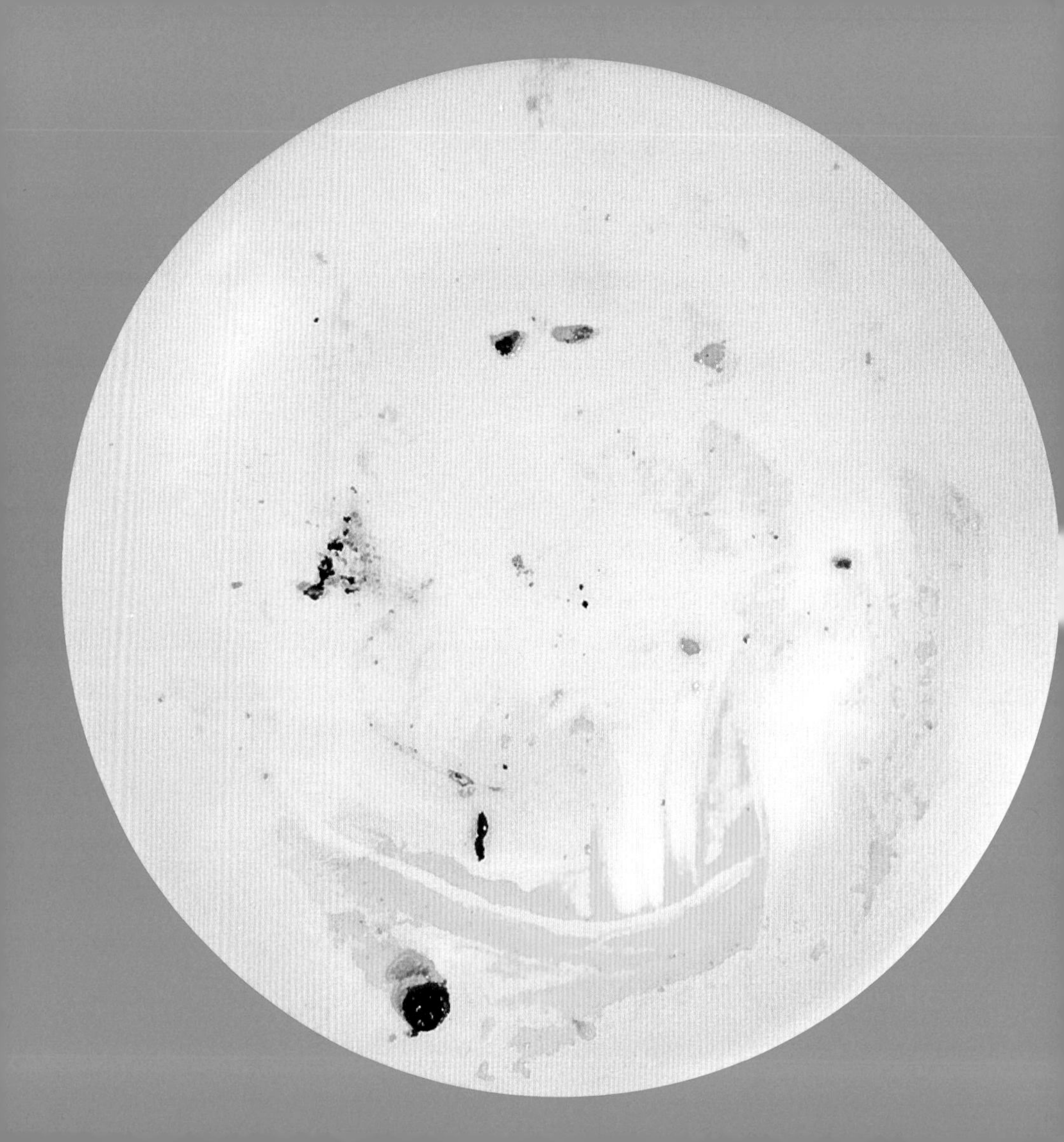

Foreword

I am not fat. Yes, I have cellulite. Yes, my thighs jiggle. Yes, I have love handles. But by today's ample standards, I am not fat.

This is not for lack of trying.

I have fried banana bread in butter and eaten it. One trip to Ben & Jerry's saw me get a waffle cone with three scoops of ice cream and, because it was there, a brownie on top of it. Bacon is not a breakfast side dish so much as it is breakfast, and I've been known to save the grease to cook or bake with later. I've even improved on the low-calorie blandness of popcorn by popping it in said grease. Thanks to a Price Club membership, my freezer is full of ice cream bars, mini quiches, and meat. Lots and lots of meat.

This is all my right as a Wisconsin native, a state that once led the nation in obesity, but has since fallen to an embarrassing number twenty-five. It is also my right as someone who worked at the Illinois State Fair for twelve years and, while there, ate more fried and stick-based foods than anyone should consume in a lifetime.

With this pedigree, you would think I had seen it all, foodwise. *I* thought I had seen it all.

This Is Why You're Fat quickly dissuaded me of that notion.

Day after day after day, Jessica and Richard posted new images of edibles that left grease marks from inside the screen. Some of the items were simply novelty-size versions of existing snacks, some were meat- and cheese-based, some were fried. All of them sent a shudder through my body. All of them made me question the existence of God. At a certain point, I had to hold my head in dismay and scream to an uncaring universe, "*Why?!*"

As a nation, we could have stopped at breakfast-sausage links wrapped in pancakes, aka pigs in a blanket, and been plenty satisfied. We had it all right there; a perfect vehicle for delivering meat, salt, starches, and syrup to the mouth, along with the forbidden thrill of Foodstuffs That Should Not Be Combined. But we kept right on going, and *This Is Why You're Fat* shows us the evidence, allowing us to wallow in the pornographic temptation without actually consuming anything we'd regret in the morning and, for that matter, for the rest of our lives.

Like you'd ever be tempted. You have it under control. You have "ironic distance" from this cholesterol parade.

I dare you to gaze upon the Krispy Kreme Bacon Cheddar Cheeseburger. I'd list the ingredients, except I already did. There's not a component that makes up one of these caloric masterpieces that doesn't glisten with sugar glaze or grease.

It's revolting. It's disgusting. As a savvy and sophisticated Internet user, you should be appalled by the thought that such a thing exists. You should laugh at the poor rube who would even come up with such a thing, let alone follow through with the idea and serve it to another human being. For some reason, you don't. On a second look at the picture, the cheese looks nearly perfectly melted. The bacon peeks out seductively from beneath the top of the donut. How clever to use a donut instead of a bun!

Clever?! Where did that come from? Surely you don't admire this sort of culinary behavior. Like Pete Townshend, you're just looking at these pictures for research! Soon enough, you find yourself craving what's in that picture. And just like any good pornography, you feel guilty for wanting it.

Try to get it out of your head. Sure, you'll see things that are just plain revolting (for me, it's anything with a fried egg on top), but you're just as likely to land on something you find just as appealing and, before you know it, you'll be running out the door to the nearest convenience store to gorge on anything spinning in a heated rack.

Before you start reading this book, go get yourself a sack of rice cakes and a bottle of seltzer. You'll stave off any hunger pangs you experience and feel better about yourself for pretending to enjoy such a sensible, low-calorie snack.

Now if you'll excuse me, I have to run about seven hundred miles.

Joe Garden
Features Editor
The Onion

Introduction

Food was once the providence of celebrated chefs and critical connoisseurs. Cooking shows featured all gourmet creations and websites displayed artfully photographed delights.

Then something changed.

Perhaps it was the desensitizing of Web culture or perhaps it was a cry for help from the food-loving public. But by God—there came a day when fancy vegetable towers came crashing down and fifty-dollar mushrooms were no longer acceptable. We wanted to see the old standbys, the carnival foods of our childhoods: the sticky mess of a deep-fried candy bar, the indulgence of a greasy burger with all the fixin's. And the bacon! Oh, the bacon!

It was the birth of the nasty-food Web trend. And it was delicious.

This Is Why You're Fat is an ode to this trend—whether seen as a commentary on North American dietary habits or a celebration of the deliciously bad—we're devoted to the world's obsession with over-the-top food.

If you're wondering whether *This Is Why You're Fat* functions as a warning or a menu, we like to think of it as a finger-wagging and high five in one.

The point is simple: *This Is Why You're Fat* is where gusto meets gastronomy. The world cooked, we blogged.

Jessica Amason
March 2009

Corn Dog Pizza

The McNuggetini

Recipe by Alie Ward and Georgia Hardstark

- 1 bottle vanilla vodka
- 1 large McDonald's chocolate milk shake
- 1 container McDonald's barbecue sauce
- 2 Chicken McNuggets

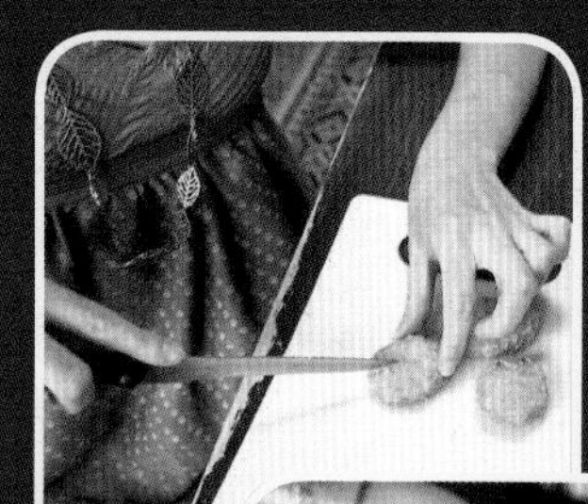

Mix 3 to 4 shots of vanilla vodka in the McDonald's chocolate milk shake. Rim each martini glass with McDonald's barbecue sauce and pour the milk shake and vodka mixture into the glass. Garnish each with one McNugget.

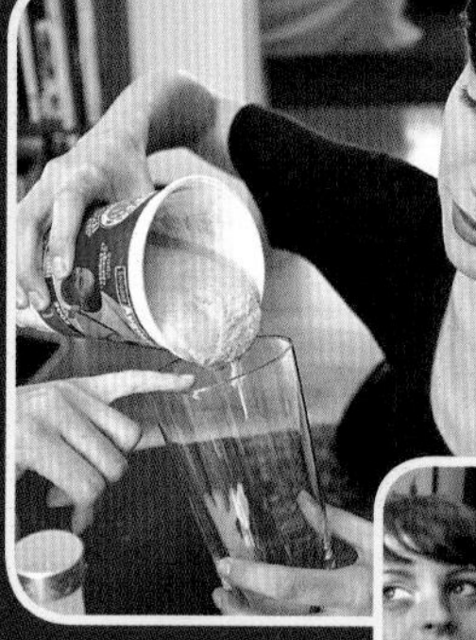

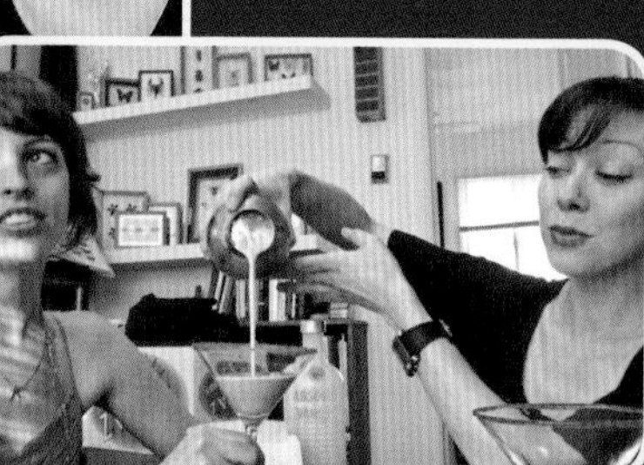

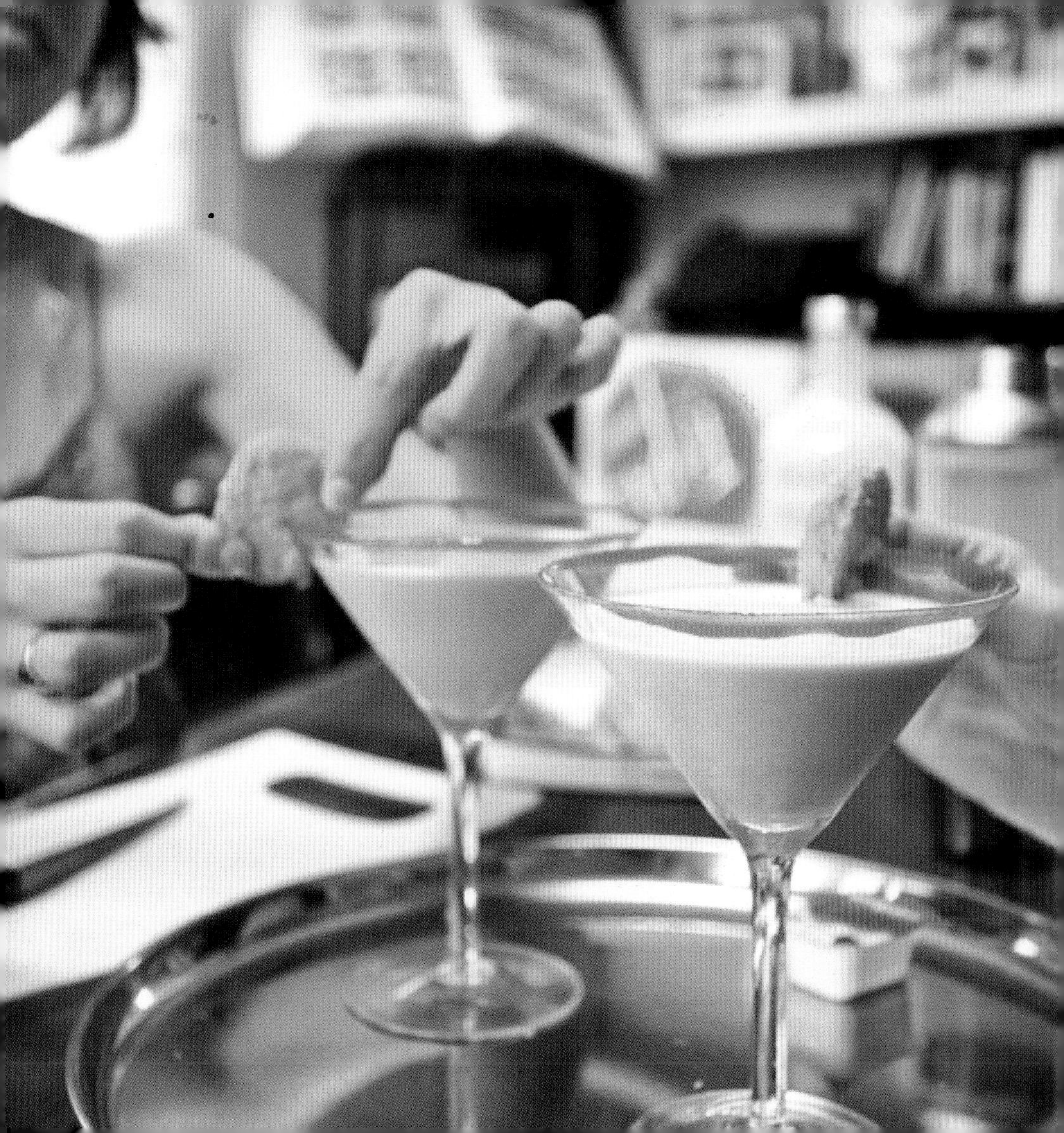

Cracklin'

Pieces of pork fat, meat, and skin, twice deep-fried.

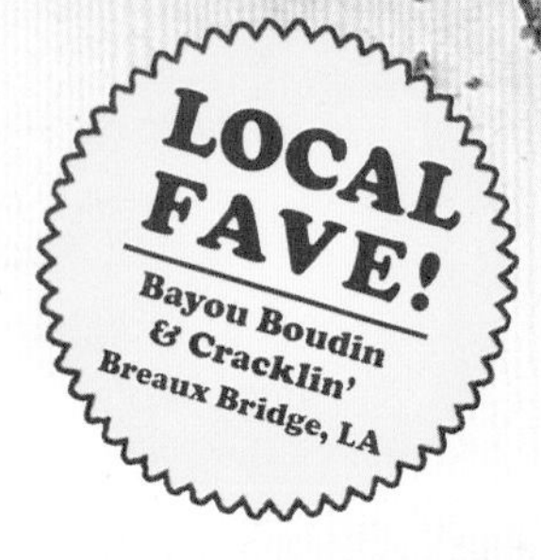

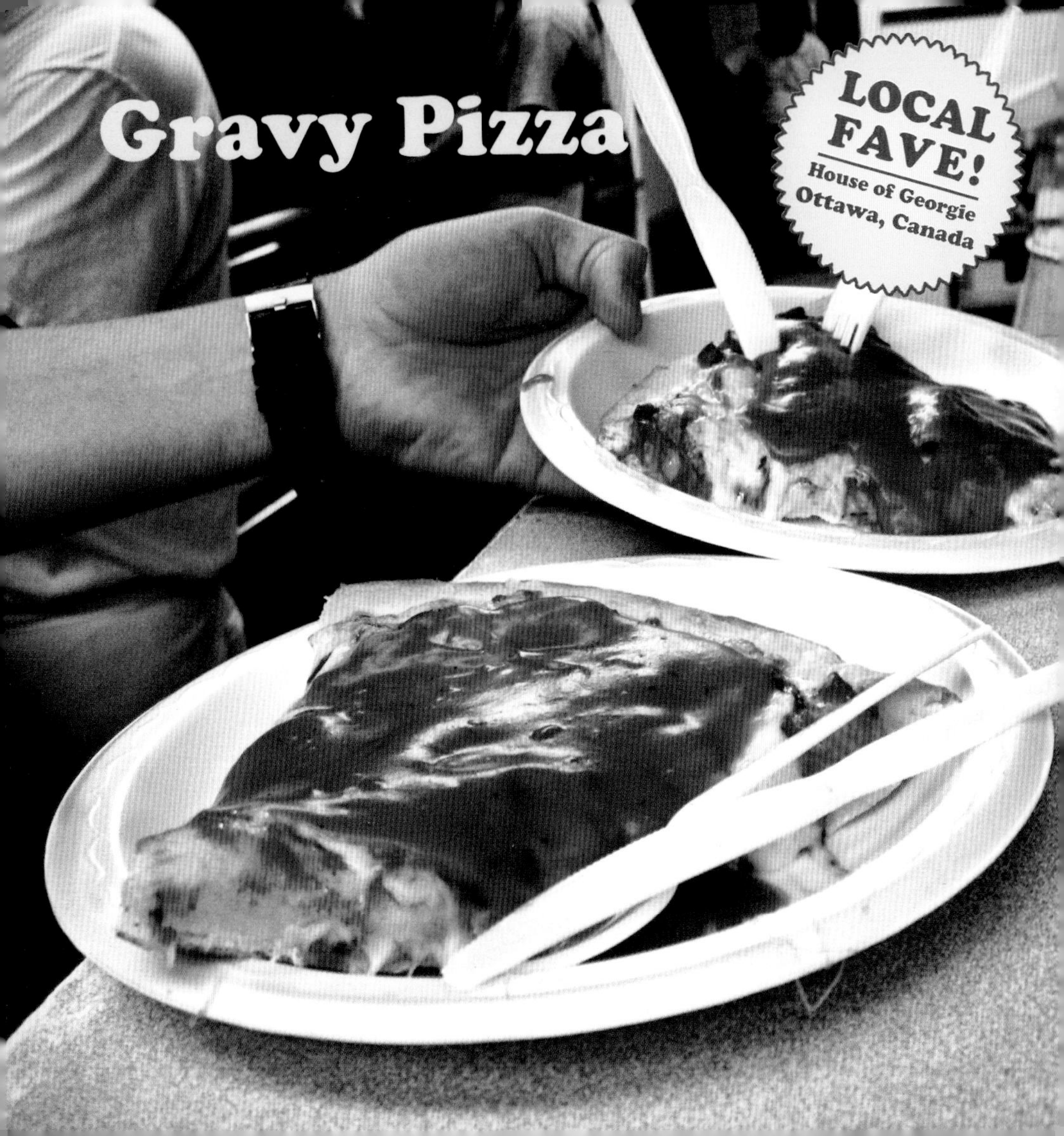
Gravy Pizza
LOCAL FAVE!
House of Georgie
Ottawa, Canada

Happy Meal Pizza

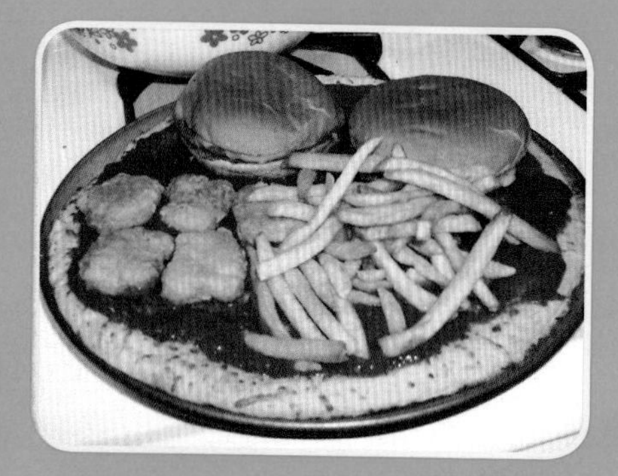

2 McDonald's double cheeseburgers
1 6-piece Chicken McNuggets
1 order of large fries
1 can pizza sauce
1 bag shredded mozzarella cheese
1 12-inch Boboli pizza crust

Cook at 440°F for 10 minutes.

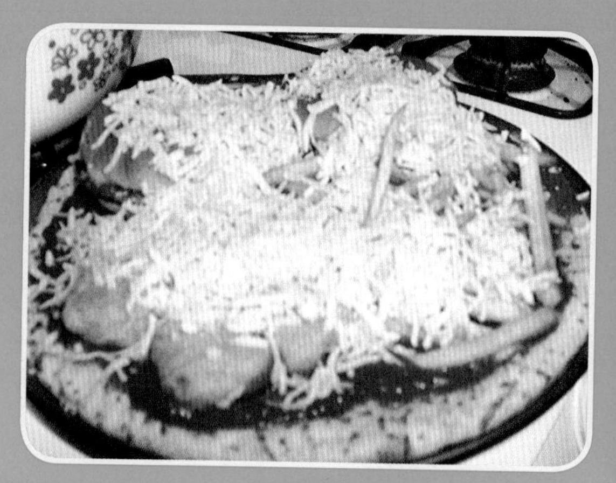

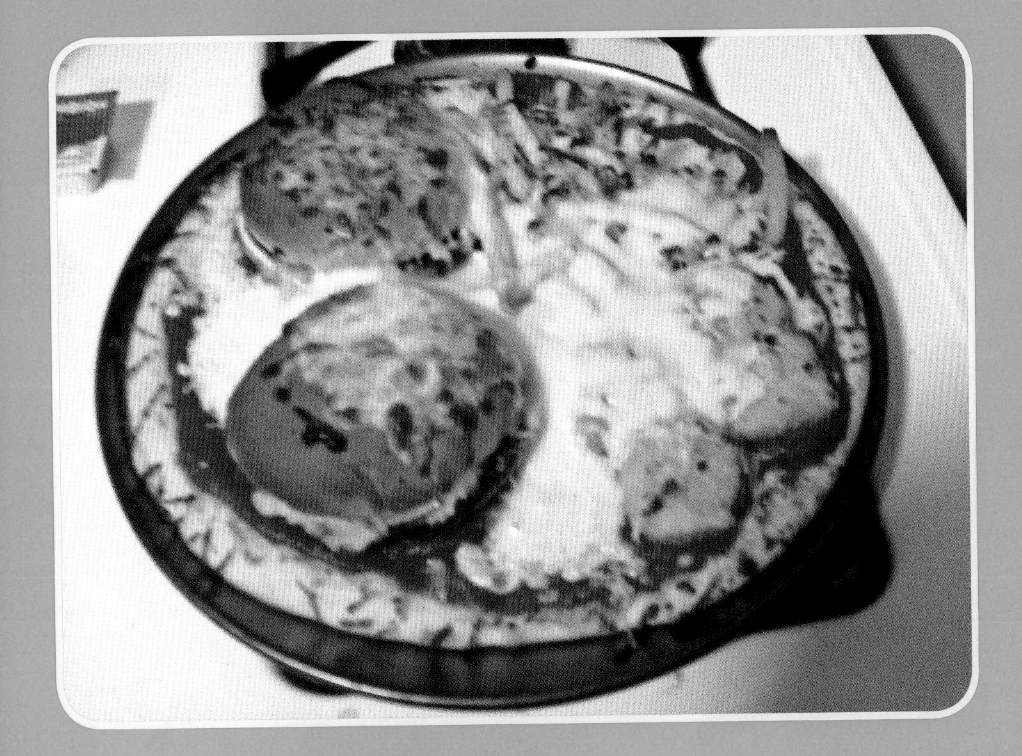

TriMacta

Deep-fried mac-and-cheese rolls on crema agria with bacon sprinkles.

Twinkie Weiner Sandwich

Inspired by the "Weird Al" Yankovic film UHF, a hot dog with a Twinkie for a bun topped with Cheez Whiz.

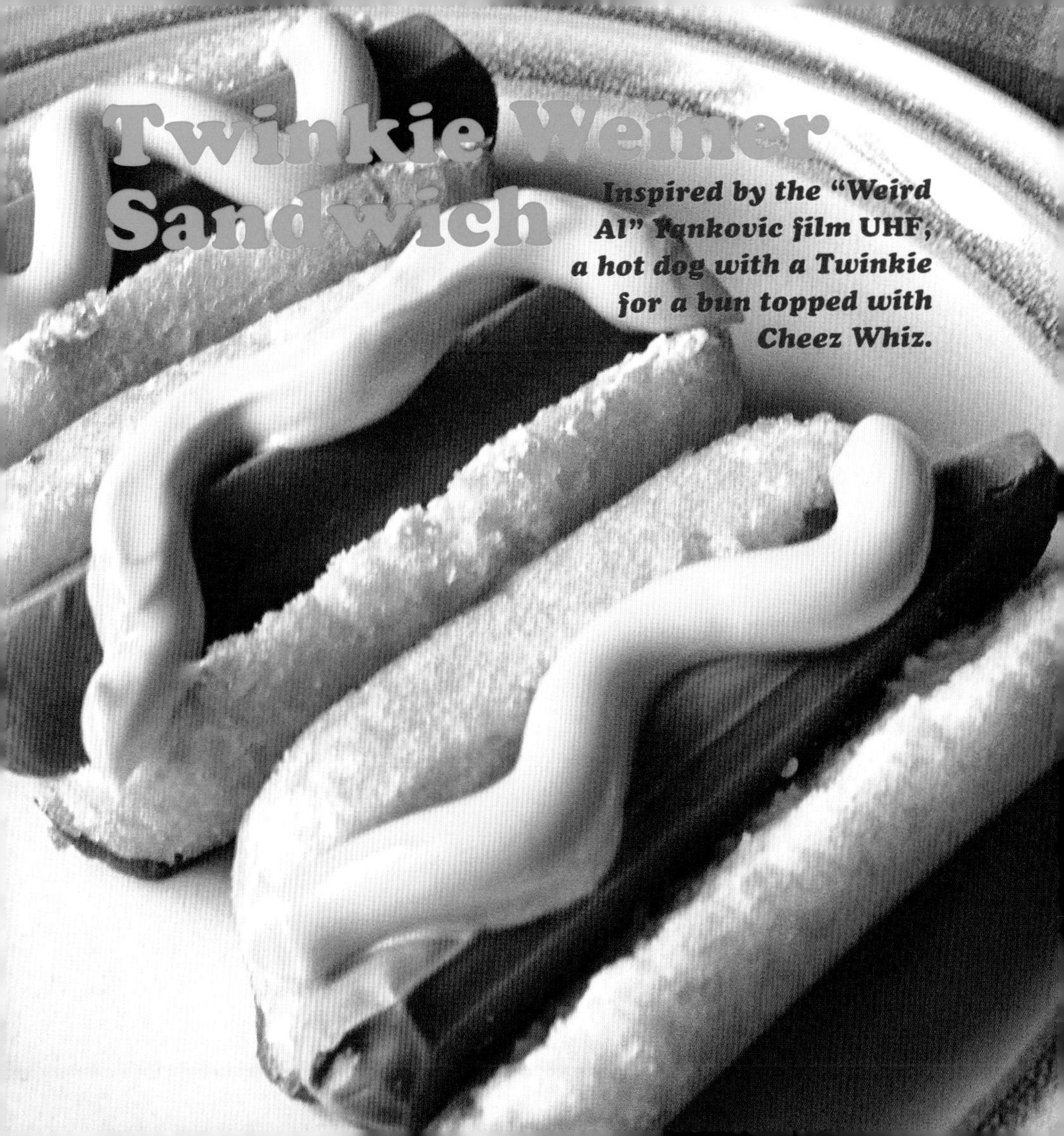

Taco Town Taco

Recipe by Doyle Dodd and Drew Sloan

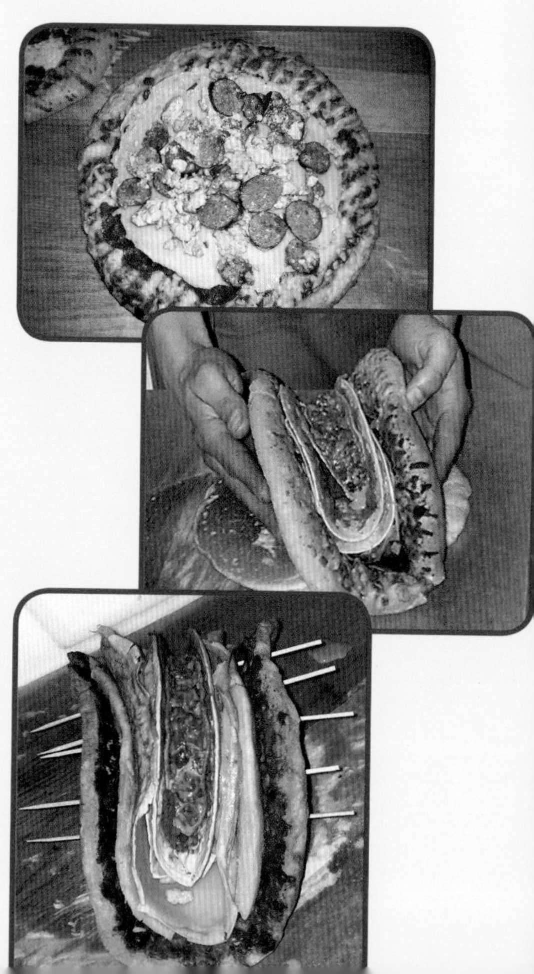

Step One:

Take a crunchy beef taco filled with nacho cheese, lettuce, tomato, and Southwestern sauce and wrap it in a soft flour tortilla, layering refried beans in between.

Step Two:

Wrap in a corn tortilla with a layer of Monterey Jack cheese.

Step Three:

Wrap in a deep-fried gordita shell with guacamole sauce around it.

Step Four:

Bake in a corn husk and top with pico de gallo.

Step Five:

Wrap in a crepe filled with egg, Gruyère cheese, sausage, and portobello mushrooms.

Step Six:

Take the whole thing and wrap in a Chicago-style deep-dish "Meat Lovers" pizza.

Step Seven:

Wrap in a blueberry pancake.

Step Eight:

Dip in batter and deep-fry the entire thing.

Step Nine:

Serve with a spicy vegetarian chili dipping sauce.

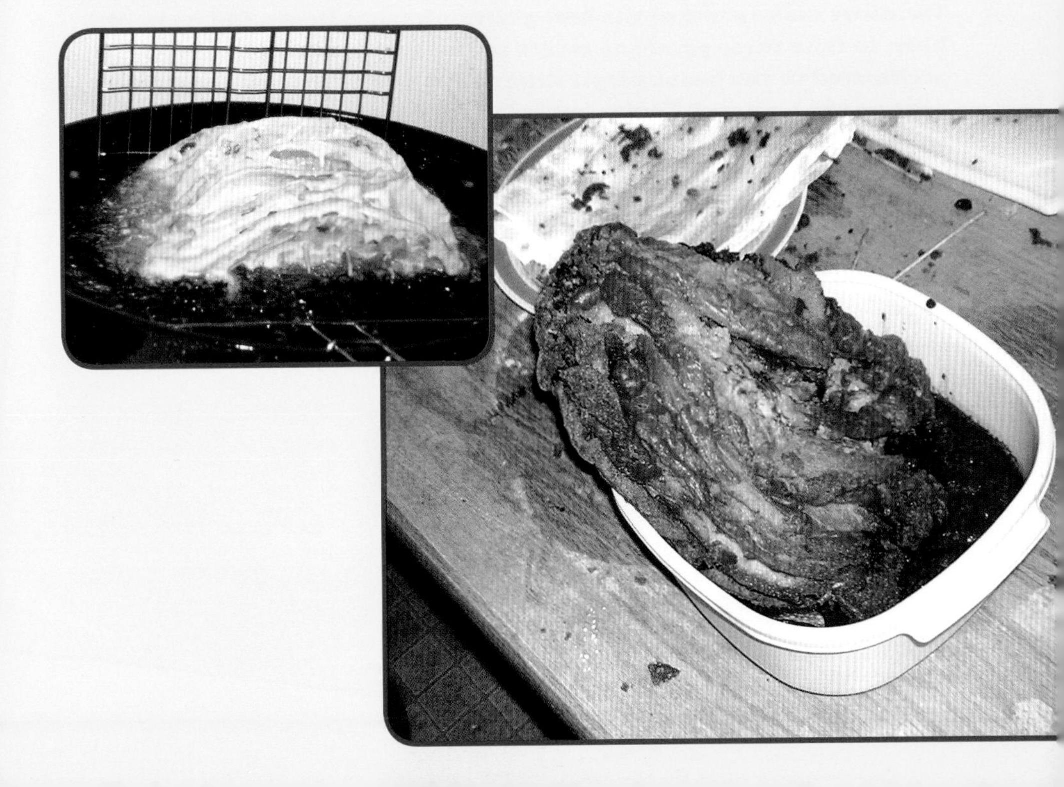

Deep-Fried Sweets

Deep-Fried Deviled Egg

Indulgent snacks like candy bars, chocolate crème eggs, and Twinkies make some of the best guilty-pleasure foods. But how, oh how, to take these premade treats to the next level? Once you've acclimated to the heart palpitations of an Oreo sugar rush, what is next on the horizon? You're left with only one solution: break out the pot o' oil and deep-fry those sweets! Oh yeah, we went there.

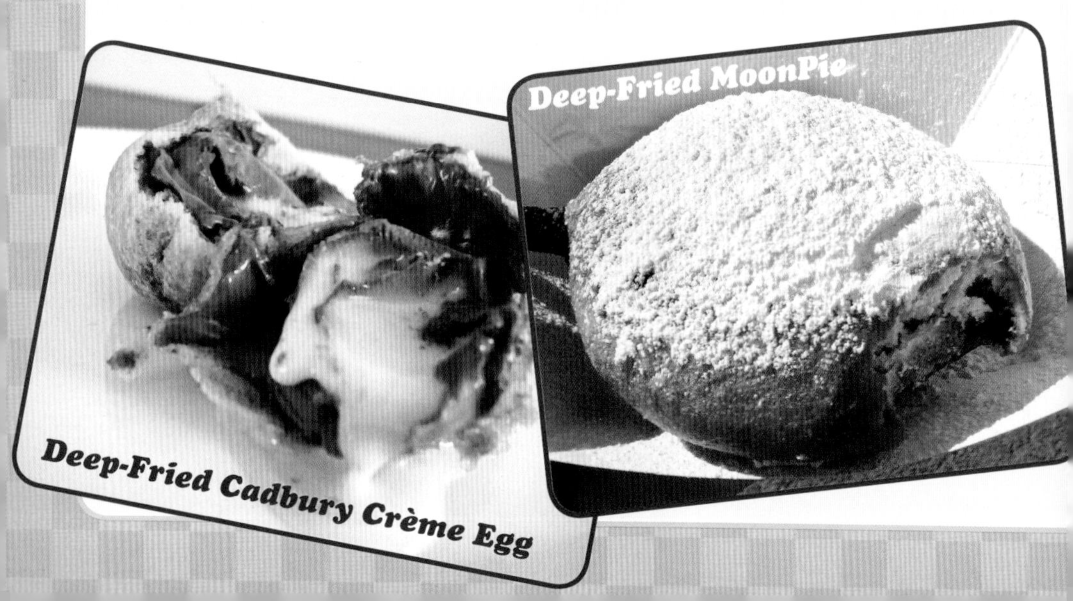

Deep-Fried MoonPie

Deep-Fried Cadbury Crème Egg

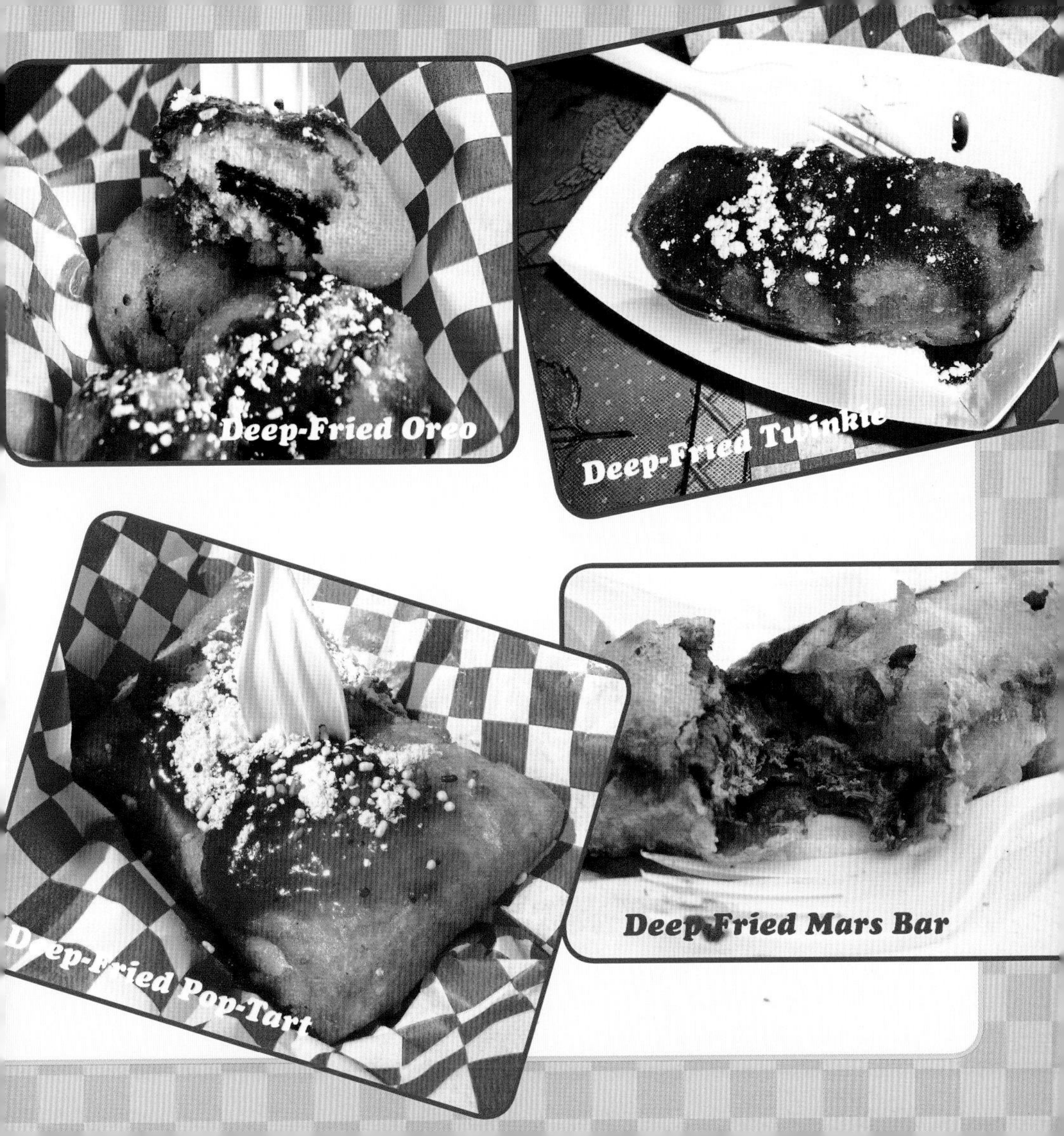
Deep-Fried Oreo
Deep-Fried Twinkie
Deep-Fried Pop-Tart
Deep-Fried Mars Bar

Cadbury Egg Nog

Recipe by Seth Porges

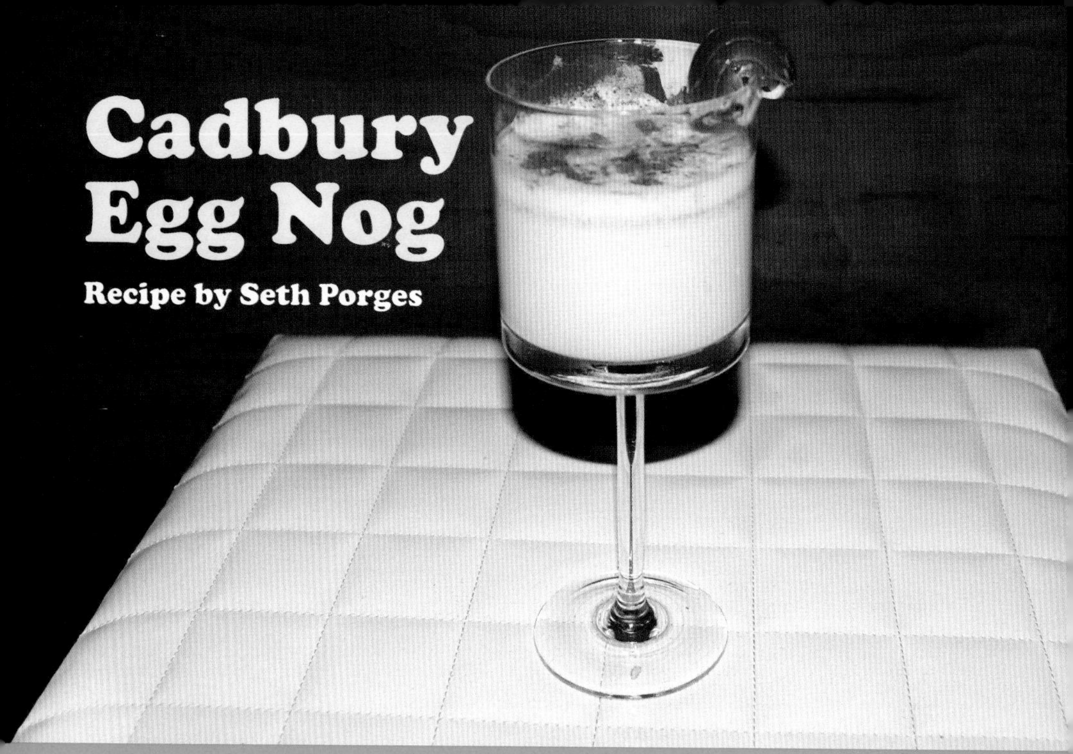

10 Cadbury Crème Eggs
3/4 cup sugar
3 cups whole milk
1 cup bourbon
1/2 cup brandy
1 tsp ground nutmeg
1 cup heavy cream

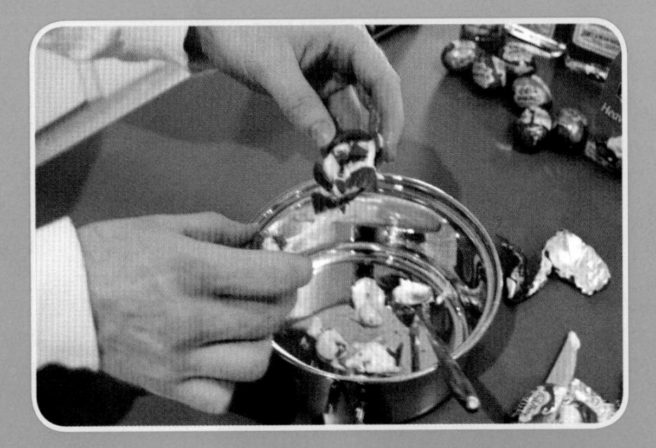

Scoop the filling out of the Cadbury Crème Eggs into a bowl. Beat the fillings together with sugar. Add whole milk, bourbon, and brandy and stir in ground nutmeg. In another bowl, whip cream until stiff. Pour the cream into the filling mixture. Gently stir. Ladle into glasses and garnish with nutmeg and Cadbury Egg shell.

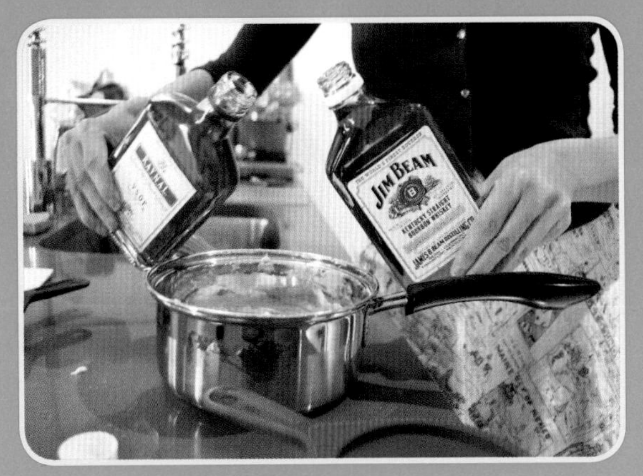

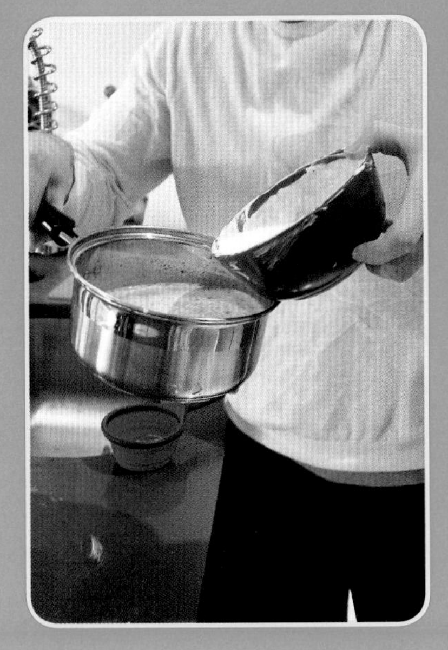

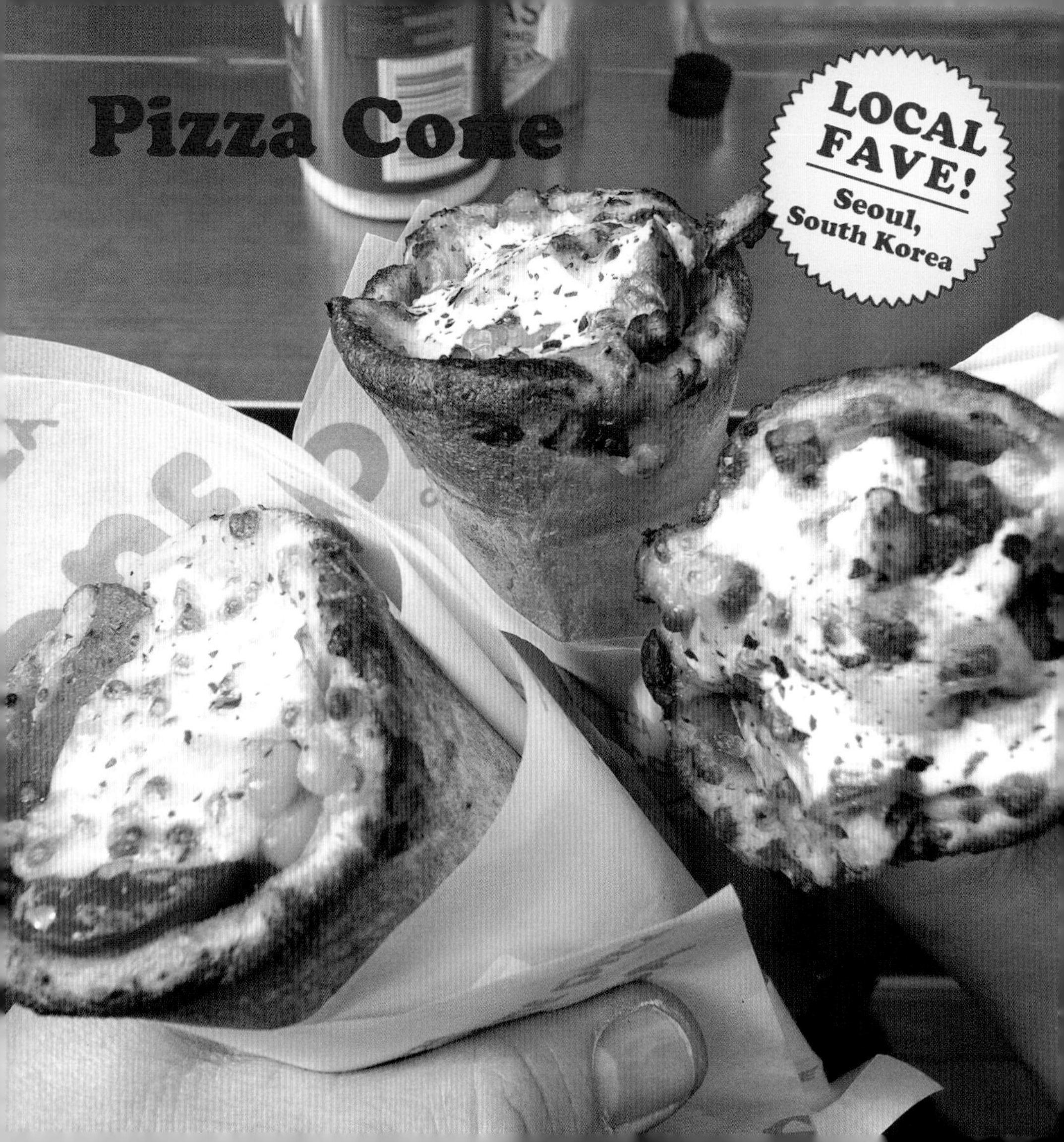
Pizza Cone
LOCAL FAVE!
Seoul, South Korea

Garbage Plate

A combination of either cheeseburger, hamburger, Italian sausages, steak, chicken, white or red hots, a grilled-cheese sandwich, fried fish, or eggs, served on top of one or two of the following: home fries, fries, beans, and mac salad. All topped by mustard, onions, or hot sauce.

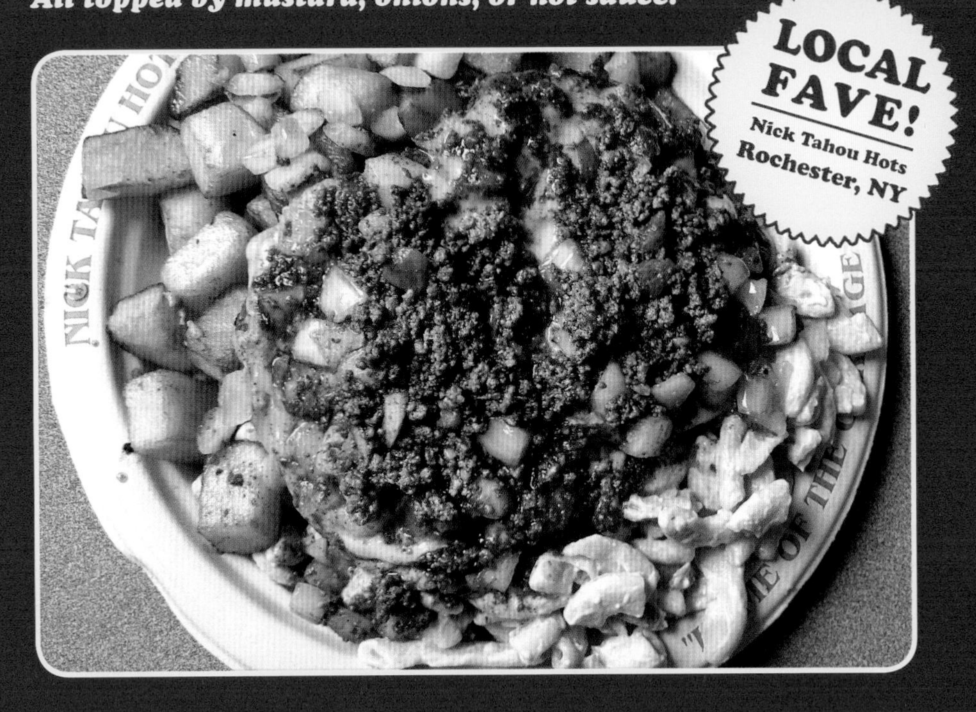

Poutine

French fries topped with cheese curds and covered in brown gravy.

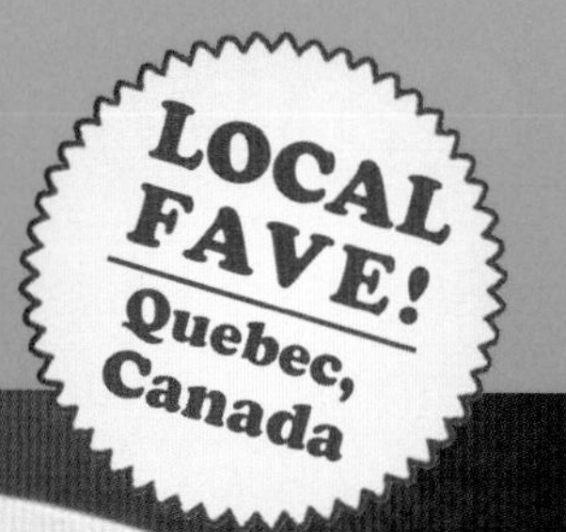

Poutine: Canada's Gift to Your Ass

BY RACHEL SKLAR (JOURNALIST AND PROUD CANADIAN)

I am a Canadian, born and bred, who has lived for the past decade in New York City—home of the Balthazar fry, the corner diner fry, that Belgian fry stand in the East Village. This city makes good fries. Yet overwhelmingly the lone fry condiment is the delicious but uninspired ketchup. Forgive me, but from a nation that put a man on the moon, I expect more. The "more" in question can be epitomized by that classic Canadian delicacy: poutine.

Ah, poutine. Even saying it sounds delicious, and a lot classier than what it actually is: French fries smothered in gravy and cheese curds. Who would not be dazed and dazzled, tempted and tantalized by a heaping plate of crispy fries, blanketed by chewy, tangy cheese, all smothered in thick, rich gravy?

Yes, yes, New Jersey, I know about your Disco fries (gravy, mozzarella, and steak fries); and yes, Texas, I know about your Tex-Mex version with cheese, ranch dressing, and jalapeños; and yes, Philadelphia, I know you've laid claim to cheese-everything. But above the forty-ninth parallel, in the wild northern hinterlands of that country that you sometimes refer to as "America's Hat," we see all that and raise you a magical blending of tastes that captures the best of the bunch, and sounds classy to boot. If this is why I'm fat, then I don't want to be skinny.

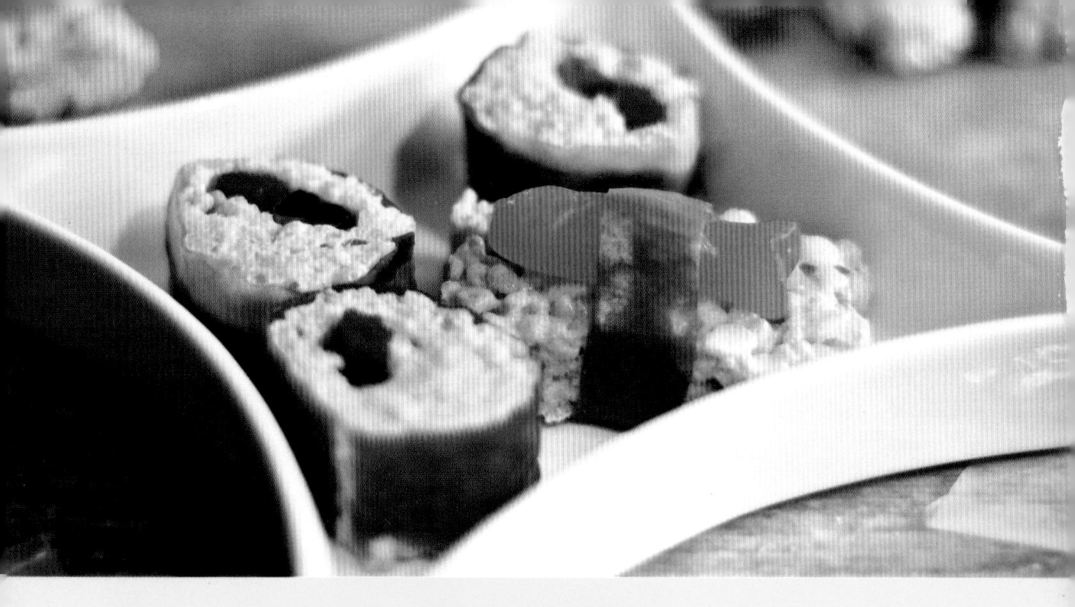

Candy Sushi

Recipe by Kim Becker

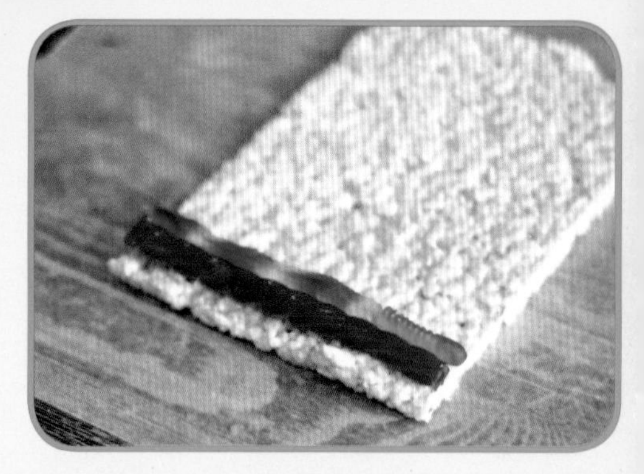

Step One:
Use any recipe to make a thin batch of Rice Krispies squares.

Step Two:
Once cooled, trim into nice, neat rectangles and stack on wax paper.

Step Three:

Add candy. In this case, colored Twizzlers, gummy worms, jujube fish, and fruit roll-ups.

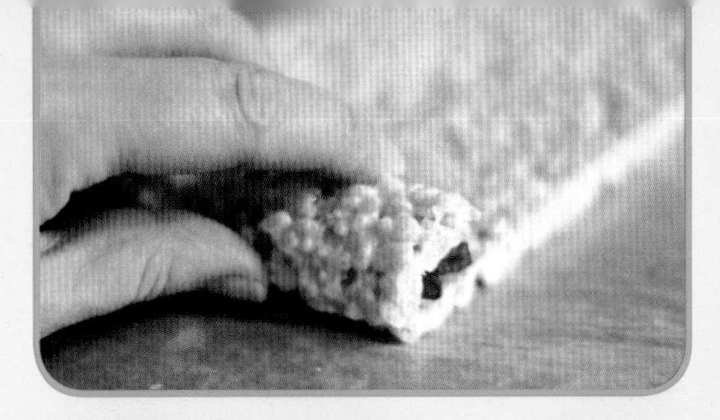

Step Four:

Roll the Rice Krispies treats around the candy. Trim the excess with a sharp knife.

Step Five:

Wrap the fruit roll-up around the roll.

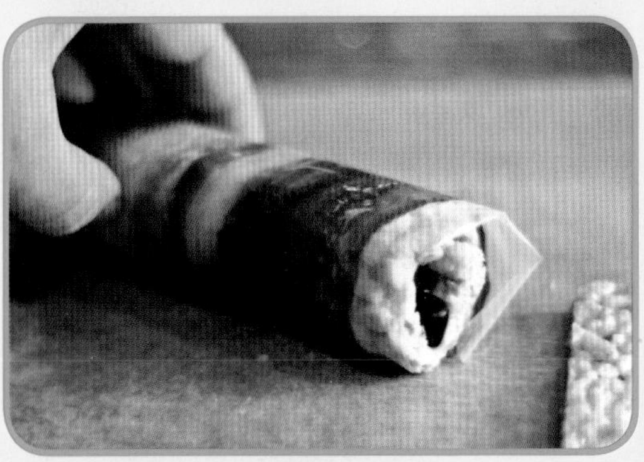

Step Six:

Cut roll into sushi roll pieces.

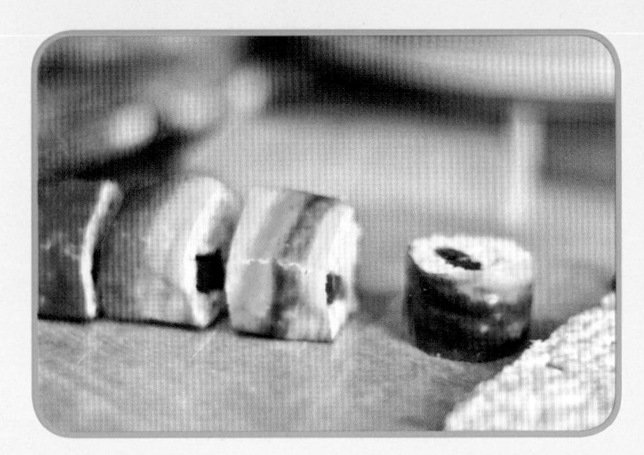

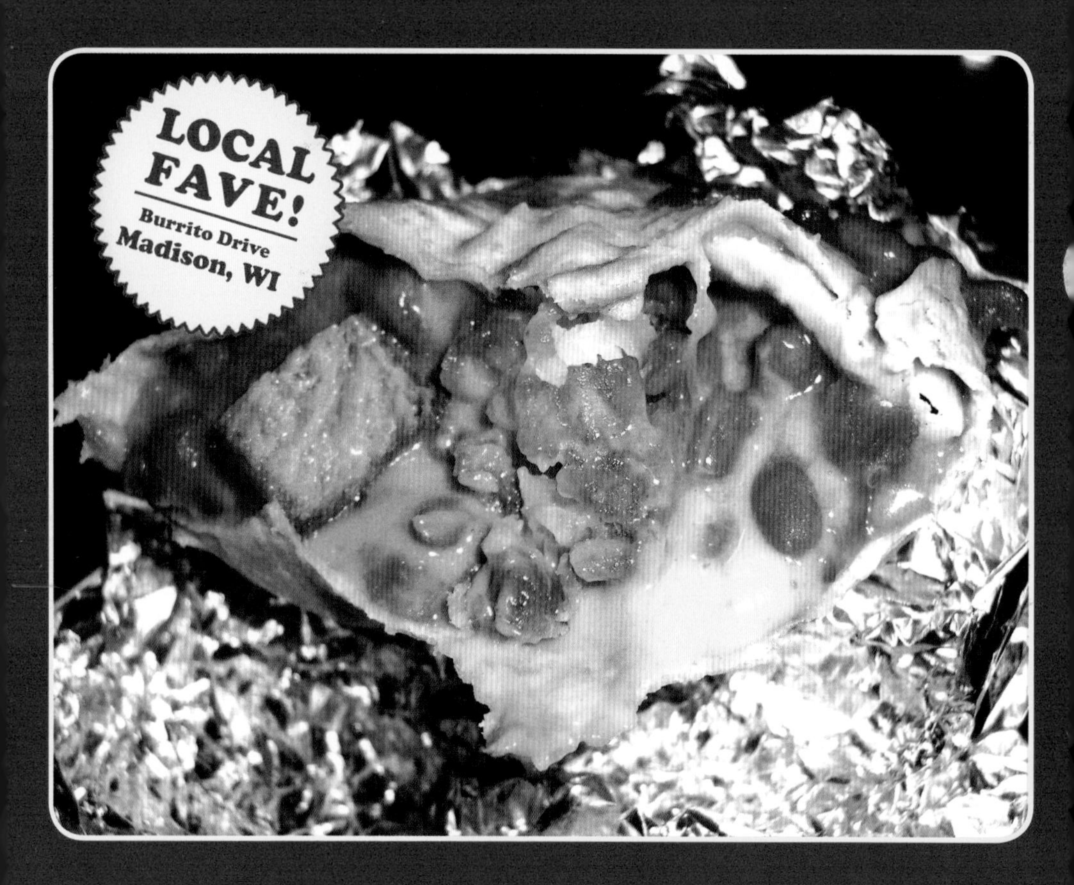

White Trash Burrito

Burrito filled with SPAM, Tater Tots, Velveeta cheese, and Boston baked beans.

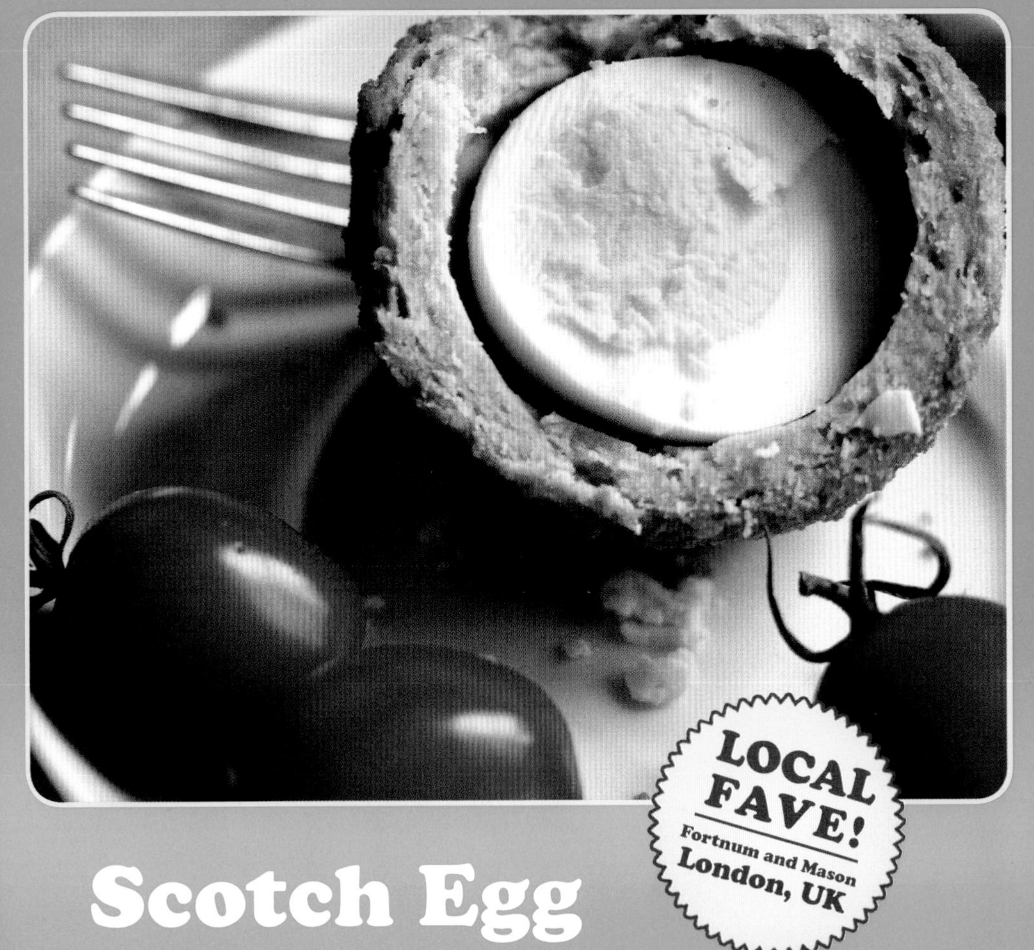

Scotch Egg

A hard-boiled egg wrapped in sausage, rolled in breadcrumbs, and then deep-fried.

Ditch Dogs

Two hot dogs topped with mac and cheese.

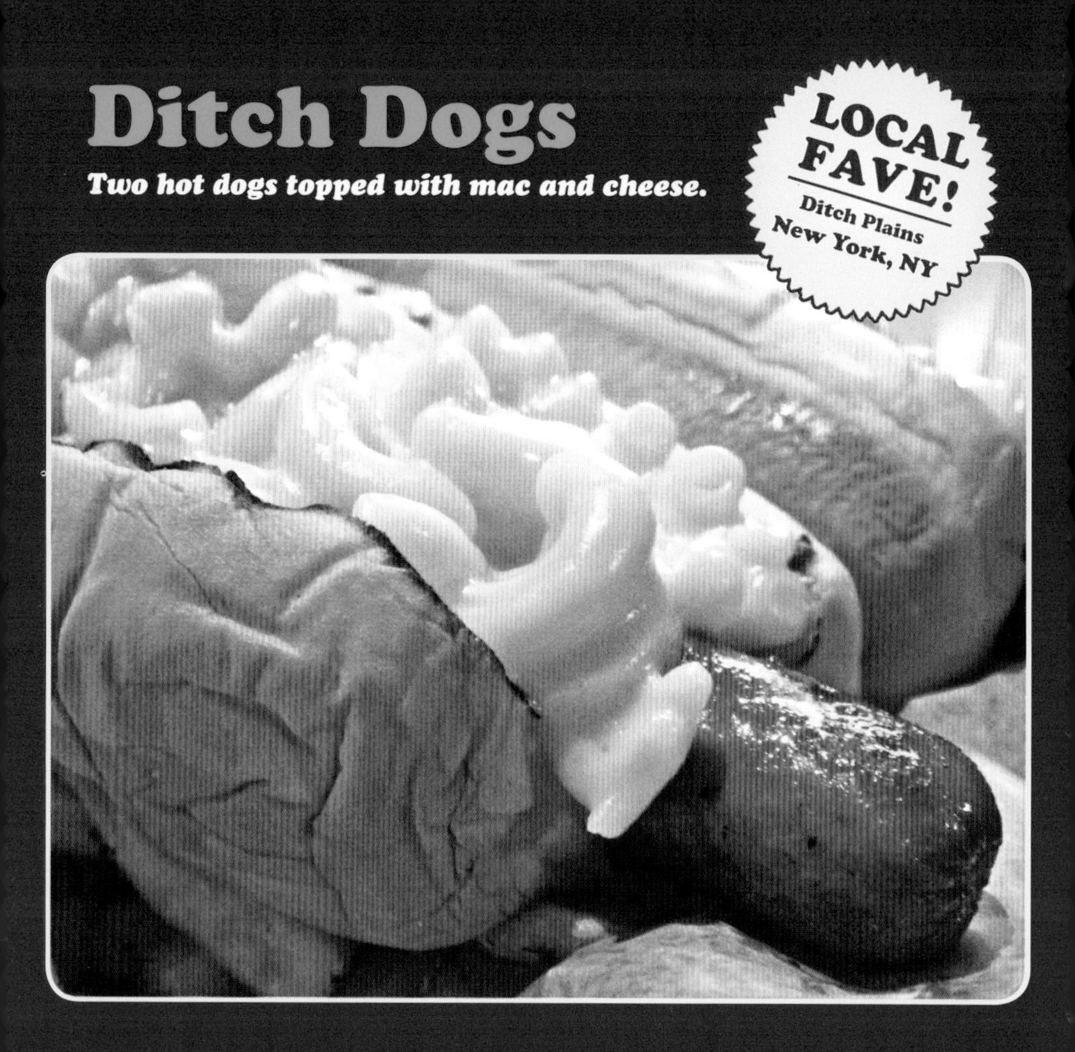

The Meatza

Hamburger crust pizza.

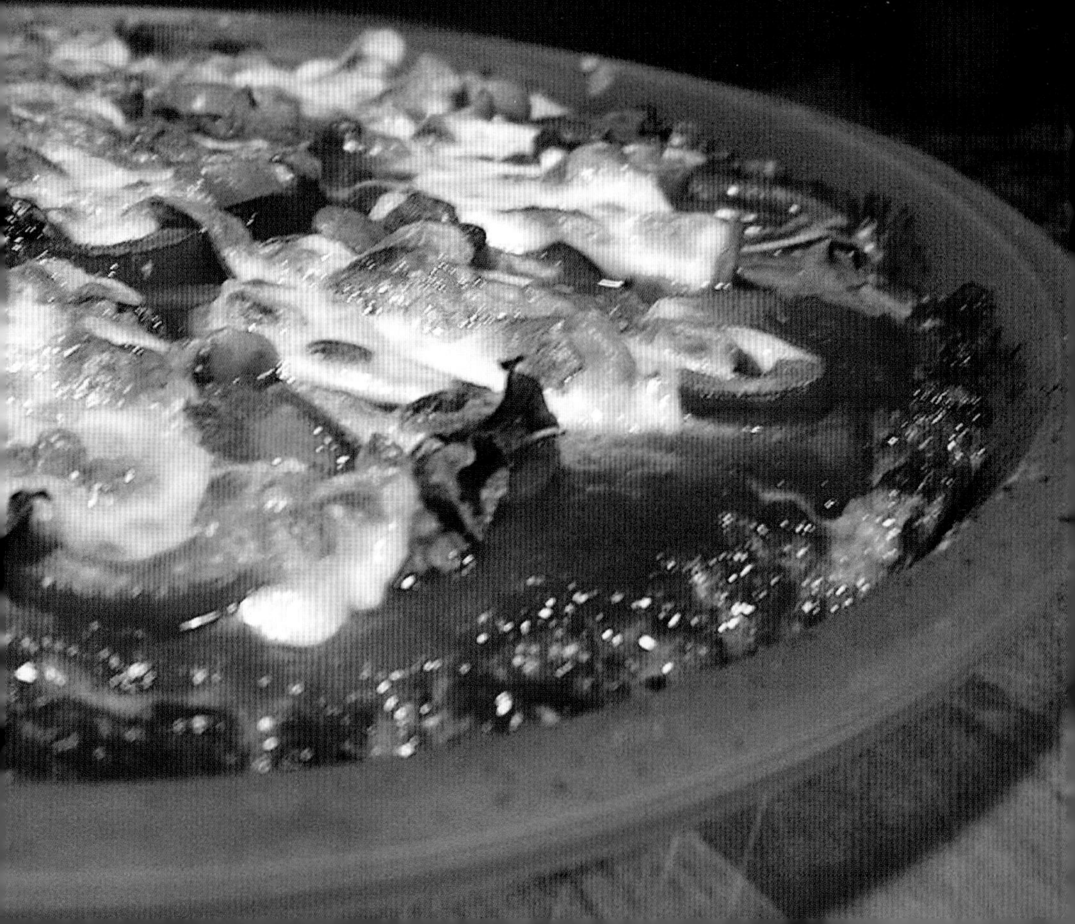

The Porkgasm

Recipe by Zach Spier and Catherine Schon

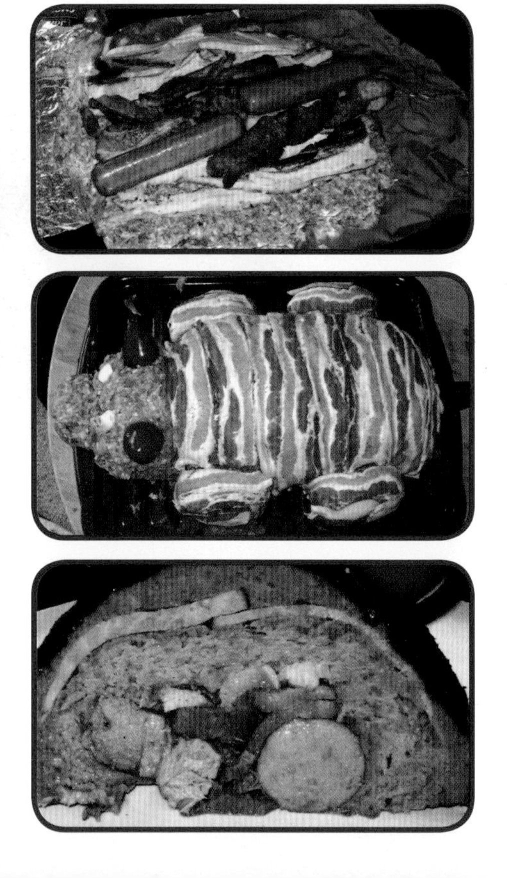

Bacon strips
Pork belly
Ham link sausage
Bacon link sausage
Smoked link pork sausage
Ground country sausage
Egg
Breadcrumbs
Salt
Pepper
Parsley
Ham slices
Ground pepper sausage
Garlic cloves
Chili peppers

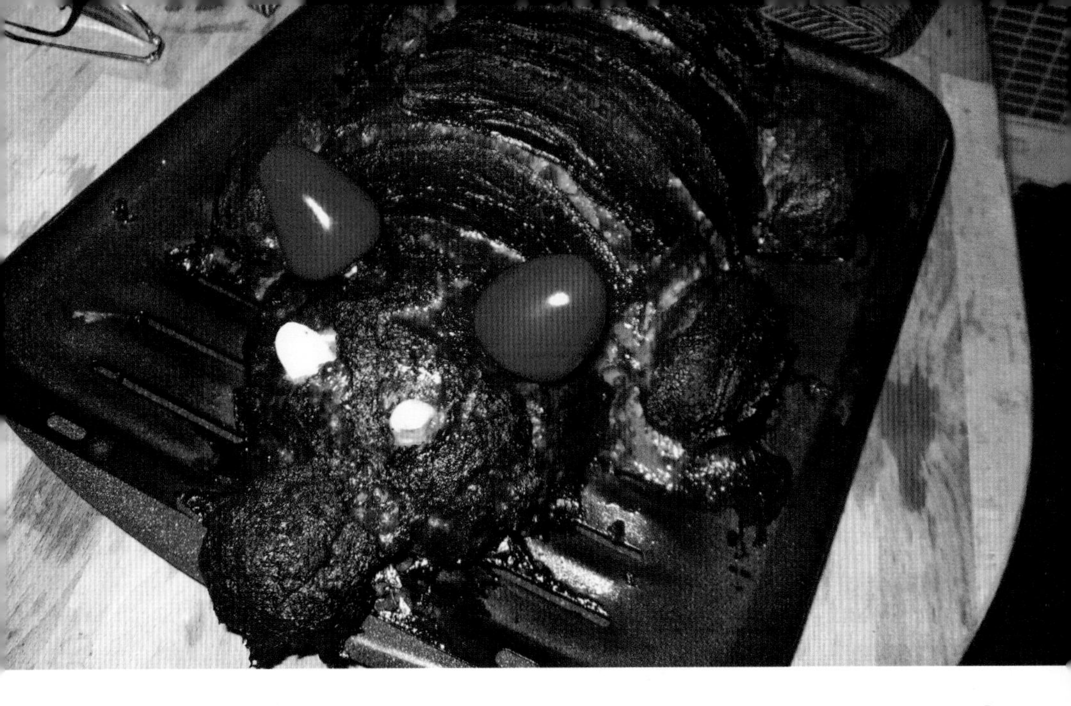

Fully cook the bacon, pork belly, and link sausages. Lay out a base layer of ground country sausage cooked with egg, breadcrumbs, salt, pepper, and parsley. Top with cooked pork belly, bacon, and link sausages, then cover the base with more ground country sausage and mold into "body" shape. Lay ham slices on top of the body. Add a "head" of ground country sausage to the body and layer all with the ground pepper sausage. Add four "legs," consisting of whole sausages surrounded by a layer of ground country sausage. Press in two garlic cloves as eyes. Layer the body and legs with bacon strips. Put the whole Porkgasm into the smoker for approximately 3 hours at a temperature of approximately 225°F to 300°F. Garnish with chili ears and tail.

Go Big!

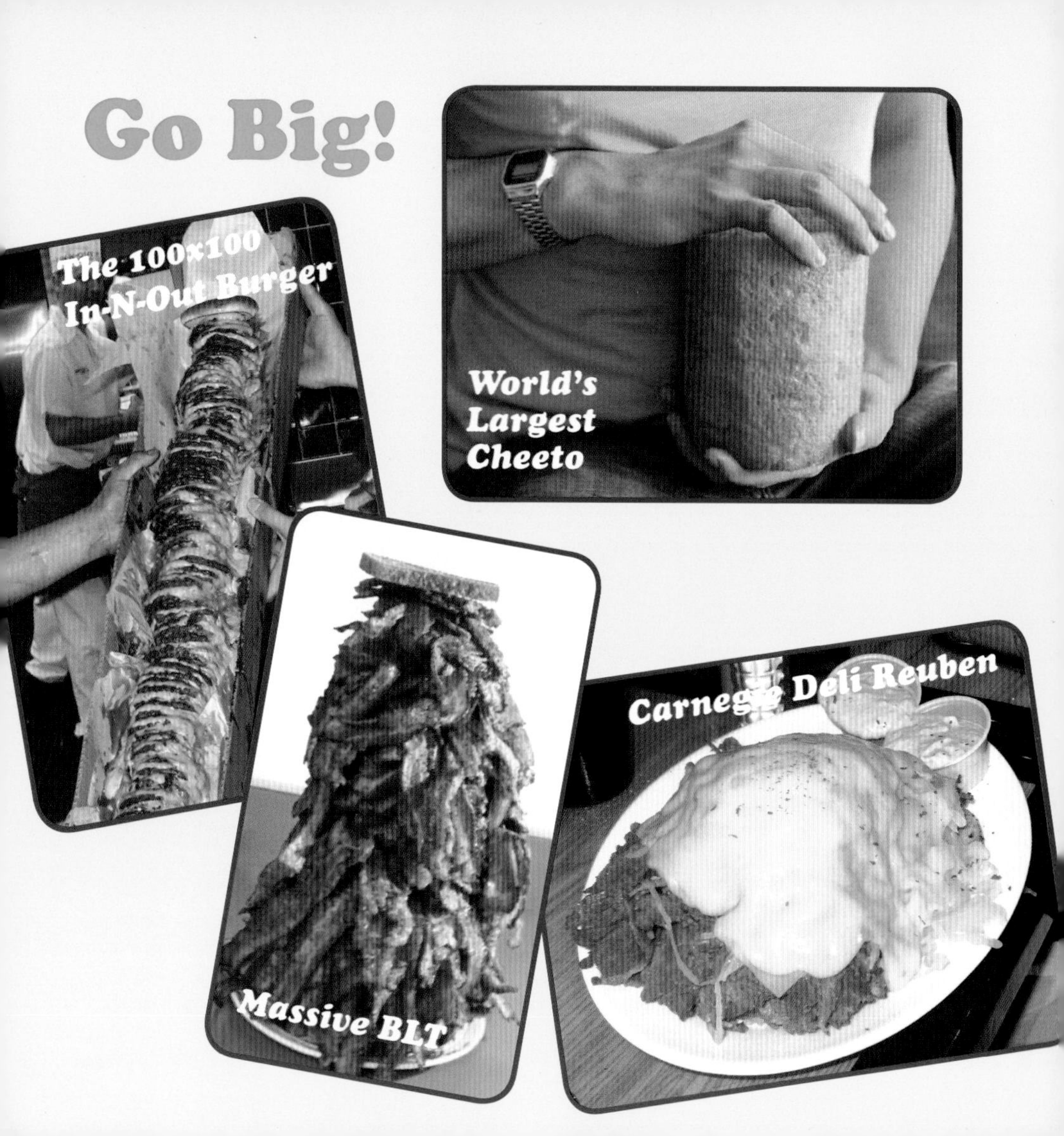

The 100x100
In-N-Out Burger
World's
Largest
Cheeto
Massive BLT
Carnegie Deli Reuben

Oversize Foods and Why We Love Them

BY ADAM FRUCCI (BLOGGER AND NOVELTY FOOD-TESTER FOR GIZMODO.COM)

Why do we love gigantic versions of regular food? One word: *power.* To hold in your hands a Cheeto the size of an infant or to settle your gaze upon a pizza the size of a swimming pool shows that you're able to harness such power over nature that you can create heretofore unthinkable objects. And to eat them? While terrifying, doing so proves that you are your body's master, able to force it to do things that are so very clearly against its well-being.

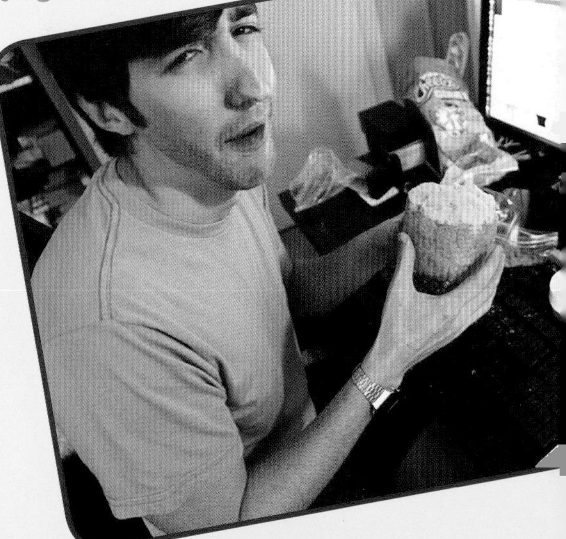

Really, gigantic food is a clear sign that humanity has reached a new peak. We no longer eat just to survive or even for pleasure. We are now so advanced that we create ridiculous-size versions of food just to prove that we can. And then, of course, we eat them. Because there's no better way to show that humans are the most powerful species on the planet than that. Until you see a koala chowing down on a eucalyptus leaf the size of a Camry, we're still kings of the jungle.

Deep-Fried S'more on a Stick

Slim Jim Shooters

Recipe by Alayne W.

Mix beef au jus, cracked pepper, and vodka, then garnish with a piece of Slim Jim.

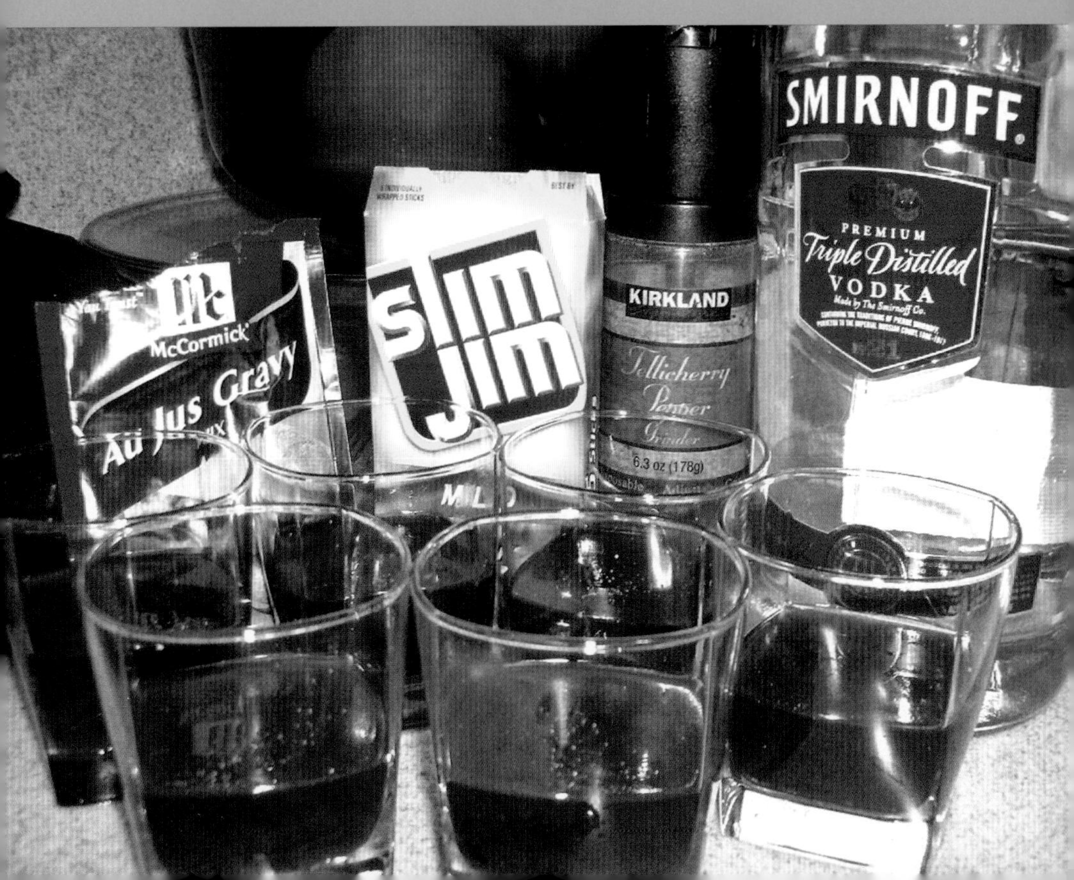

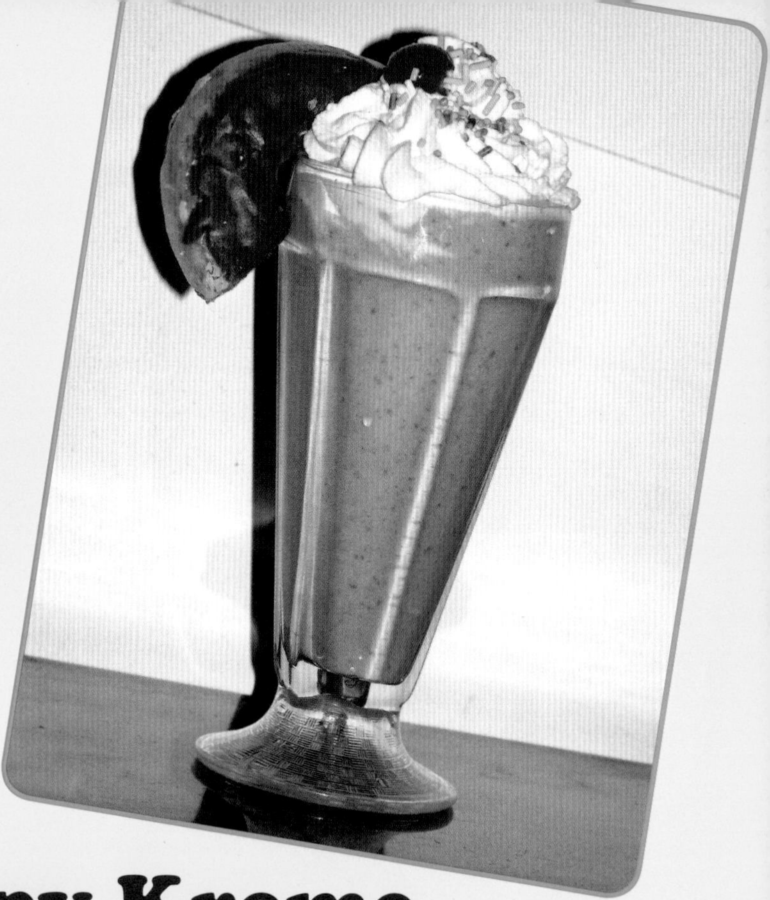

Krispy Kreme Milk Shake

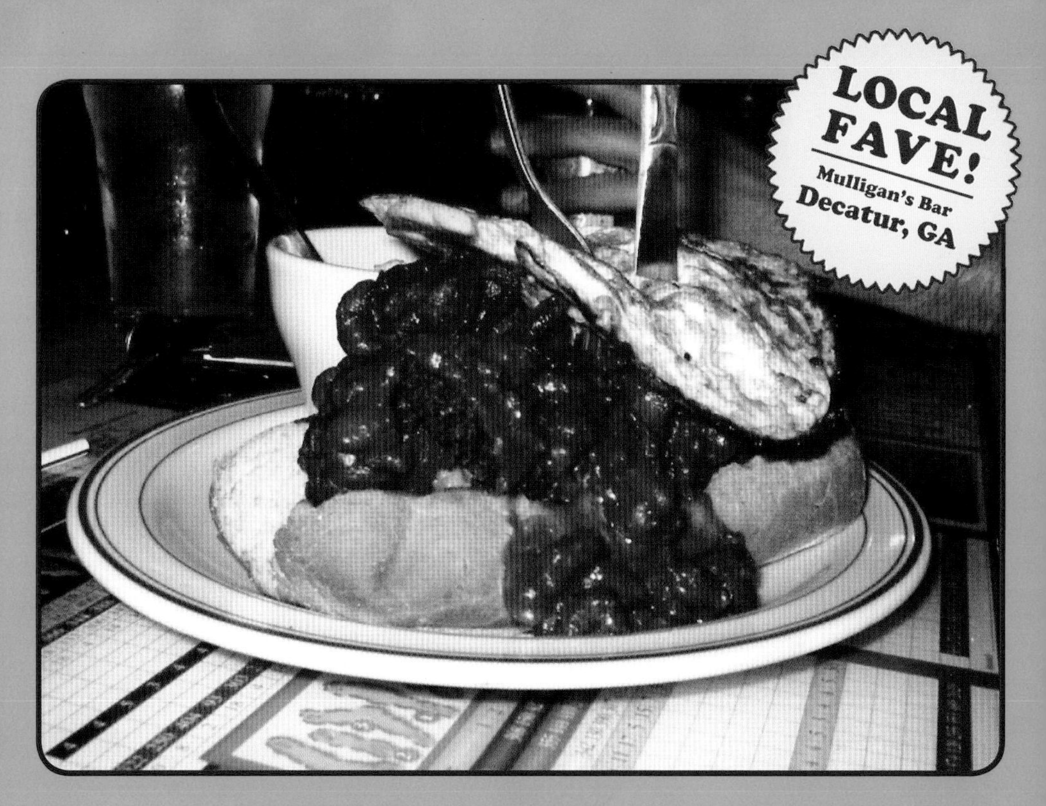

Hamdog

A hot dog wrapped in a beef patty that's deep-fried; covered with chili, cheese, and onions; served on a hoagie bun; topped with two fistfuls of fries plus a fried egg.

Grilled Cheesecake Sandwich

Recipe by Jessie of CakeSpy.com

2 slices pound cake, buttered on the outside
1 small sliver cheesecake

Assemble the sandwich as follows: Place one slice of pound cake on plate with butter side down. Place a sliver of cheesecake on top, then place the other slice of pound cake on top with buttered side up. Put in a saucepan

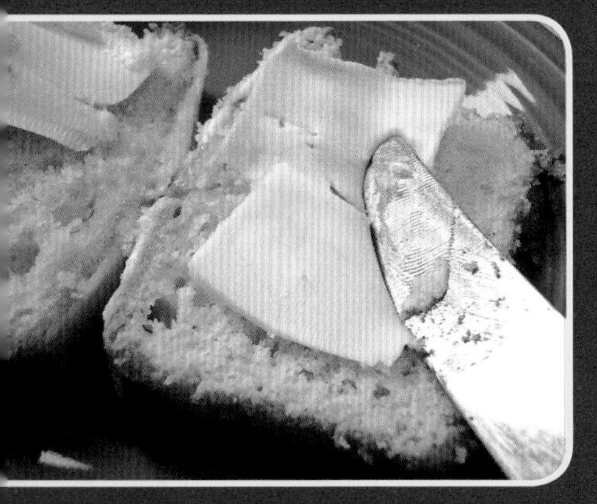

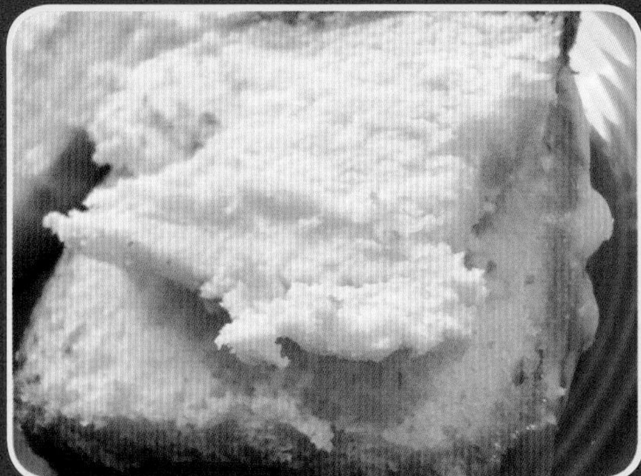

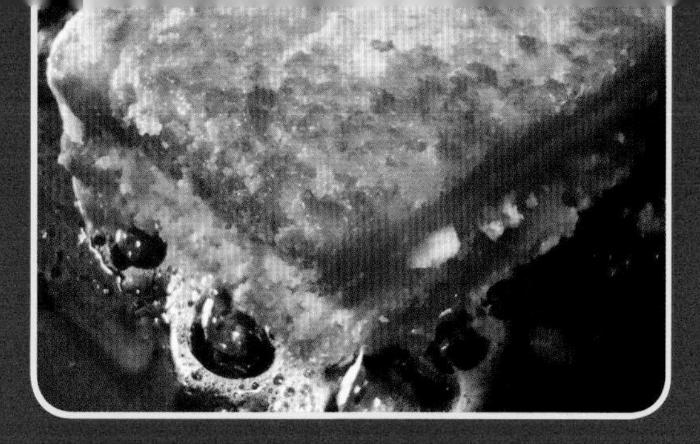

over medium-low heat. After about 1½ minutes (when browned on the bottom), flip and let other side brown, slightly pressing down with a spatula to meld together. Remove from heat, slice in half, and enjoy.

Turducken

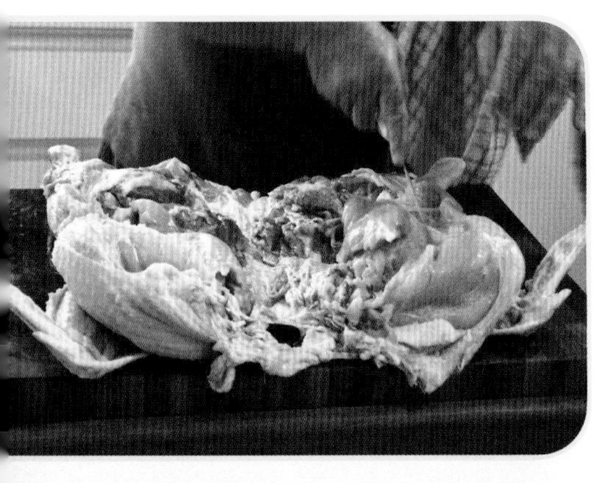

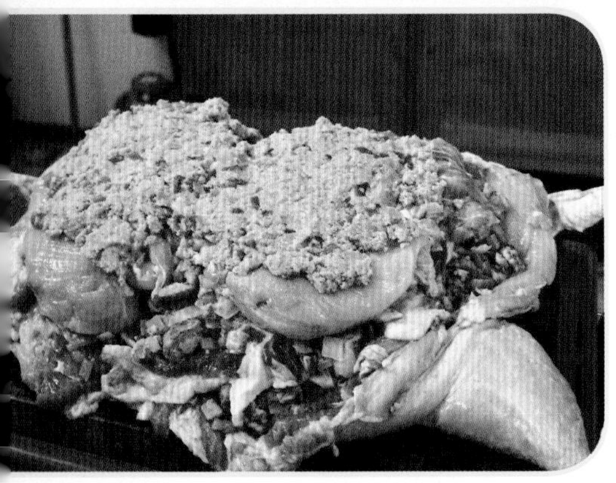

1 20-lb turkey
1 5-lb duck
1 3-lb chicken
2 loaves of bread
6 large onions, diced
2 bunches of celery, diced
3 large capsicum, diced
1 jar whole-berry cranberry sauce
17 oz walnuts, chopped
1 package of corn bread mix
33 oz vegetable stock
4 sticks of butter
Various spices
Roast seasoning
Roasting twine

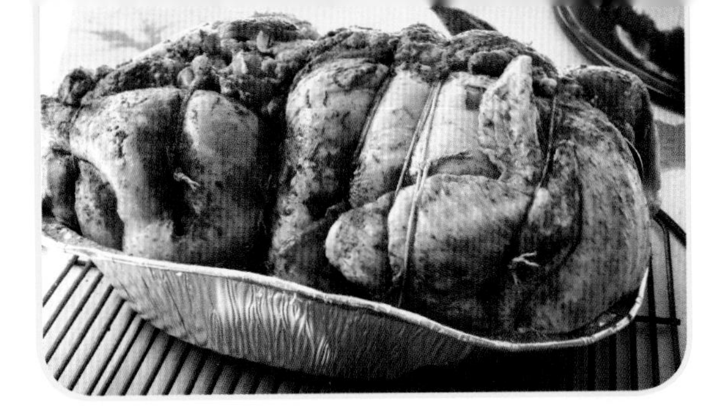

Prepare three different types of stuffing the night before; one for each layer. This recipe uses corn bread, cajun, and cranberry-and-walnut types of stuffing. Debone each of the birds, making sure that they are completely thawed first. Lay the turkey with its insides facing up and spread an inch or so of the first stuffing over it. Then lay the deboned duck on top of the turkey, and repeat with the second stuffing. Finally, lay out the chicken and cover with the last type of stuffing. Form the turducken by bringing the sides of the turkey back together and then tie them in place. Cook 45 to 50 minutes per pound, or to when the inside reaches 180°F. Season to taste.

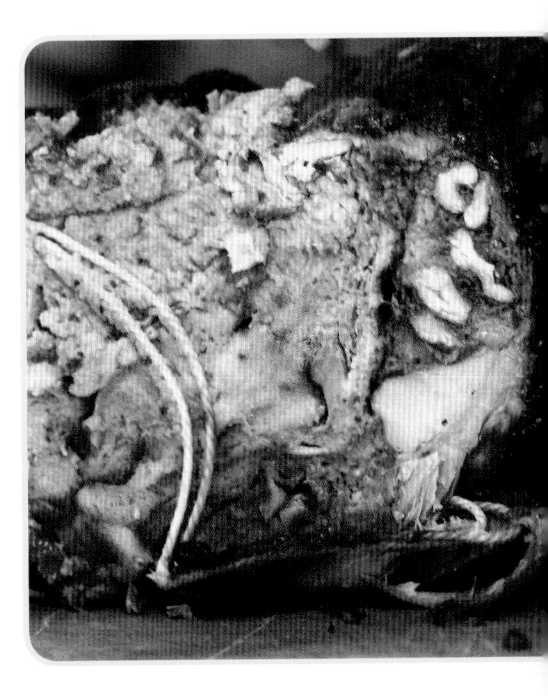

The Pizza Hut Double Roll Pizza

A pizza with a pigs-in-a-blanket crust. The center is filled with Italian sausage, ham, bacon, bacon bits, sliced tomatoes, mushrooms, onions, peppers, garlic chips, basil, black pepper, and tomato sauce.

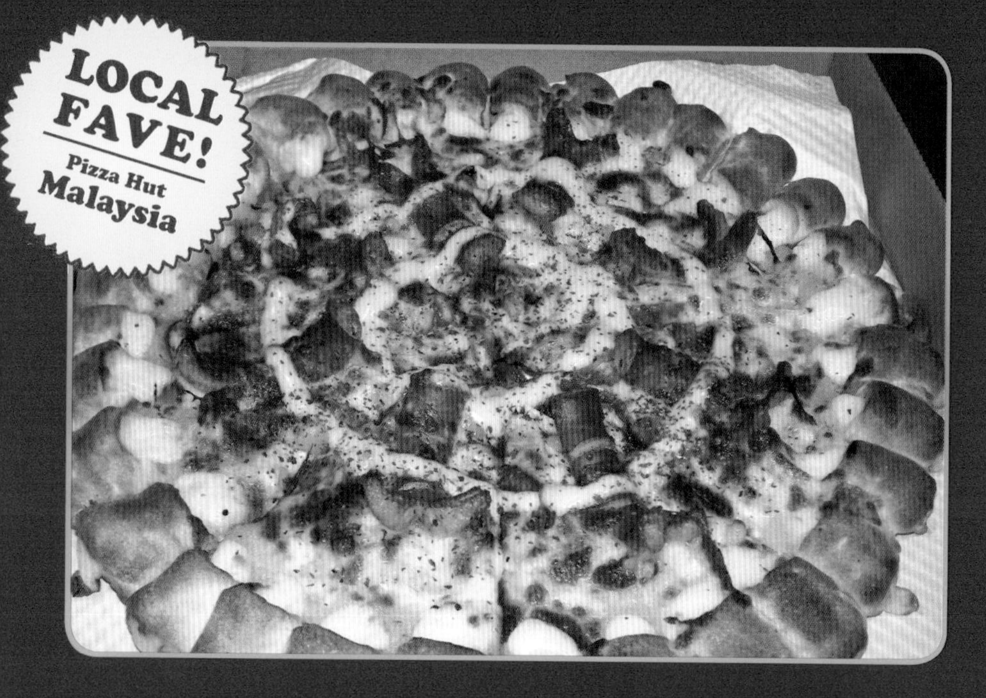

Loco Moco

A bed of rice topped with a large burger patty topped with a fried egg covered in brown gravy.

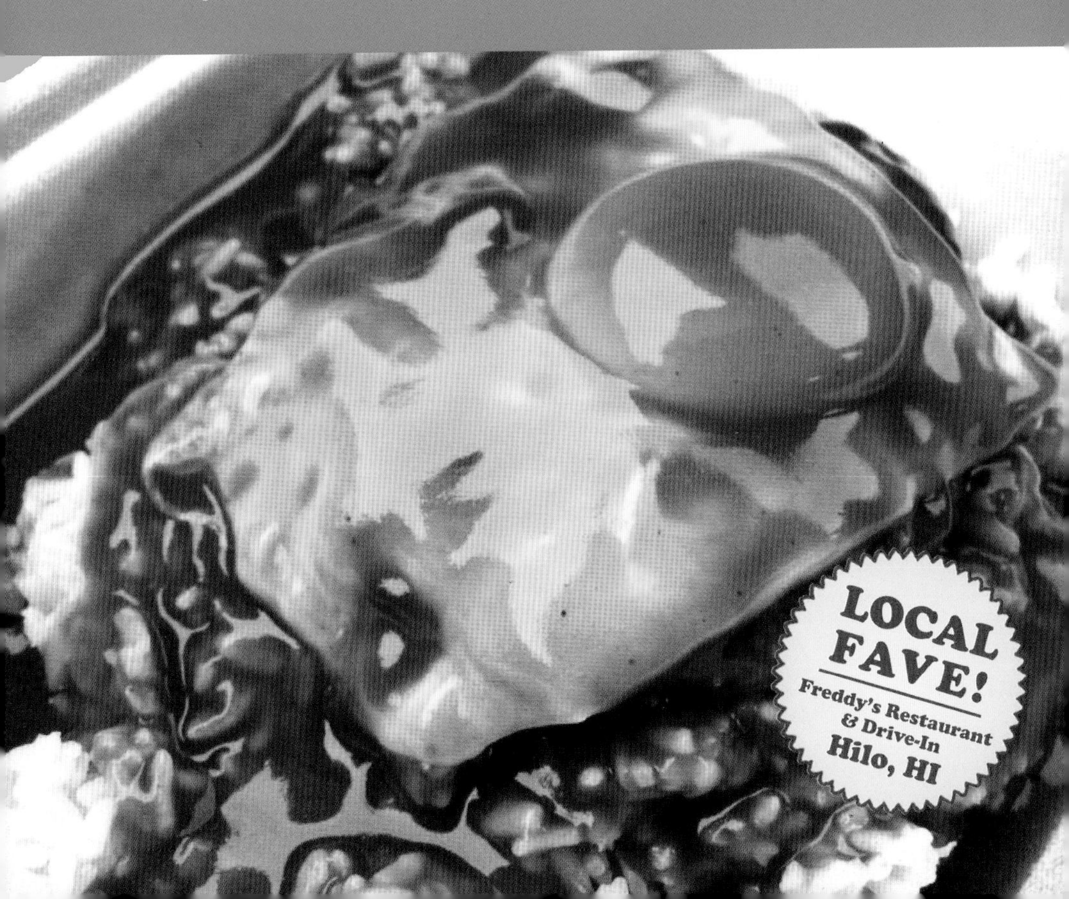

Meatabulous!

The Meat House started as a joke about whether it was possible to create a house or a structure out of meat only. I originally thought it would live and die as a funny idea, however, my flatmate—a mechanical engineer—took the challenge 100 percent seriously. First we decided to start small with a meat-based version of a ginger bread house. After a bit of planning, we gathered numerous meaty supplies, construction assistants, project mangers, and schematics and embarked upon the project. After numerous hours of planning, construction, and cooking, we were content with our greasy meat masterpiece.

However, our complacency didn't last long—soon we decided to follow up the meat house with something more complex. Various ideas were considered but we finally decided upon a meat ship, complete with bacon sails, pirates, canons and a kraken, all in a sea of blue pork. Needless to say, we'll never view meat the same way again.

—JOEL RICHARDS (CREATOR OF THE MEAT HOUSE AND MEAT SHIP)

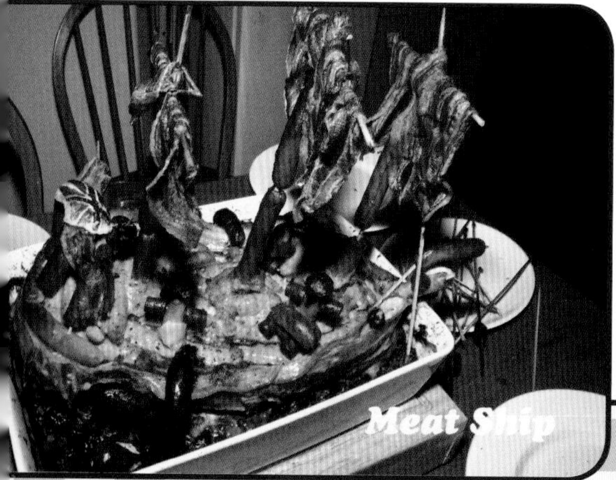

Meat Ship

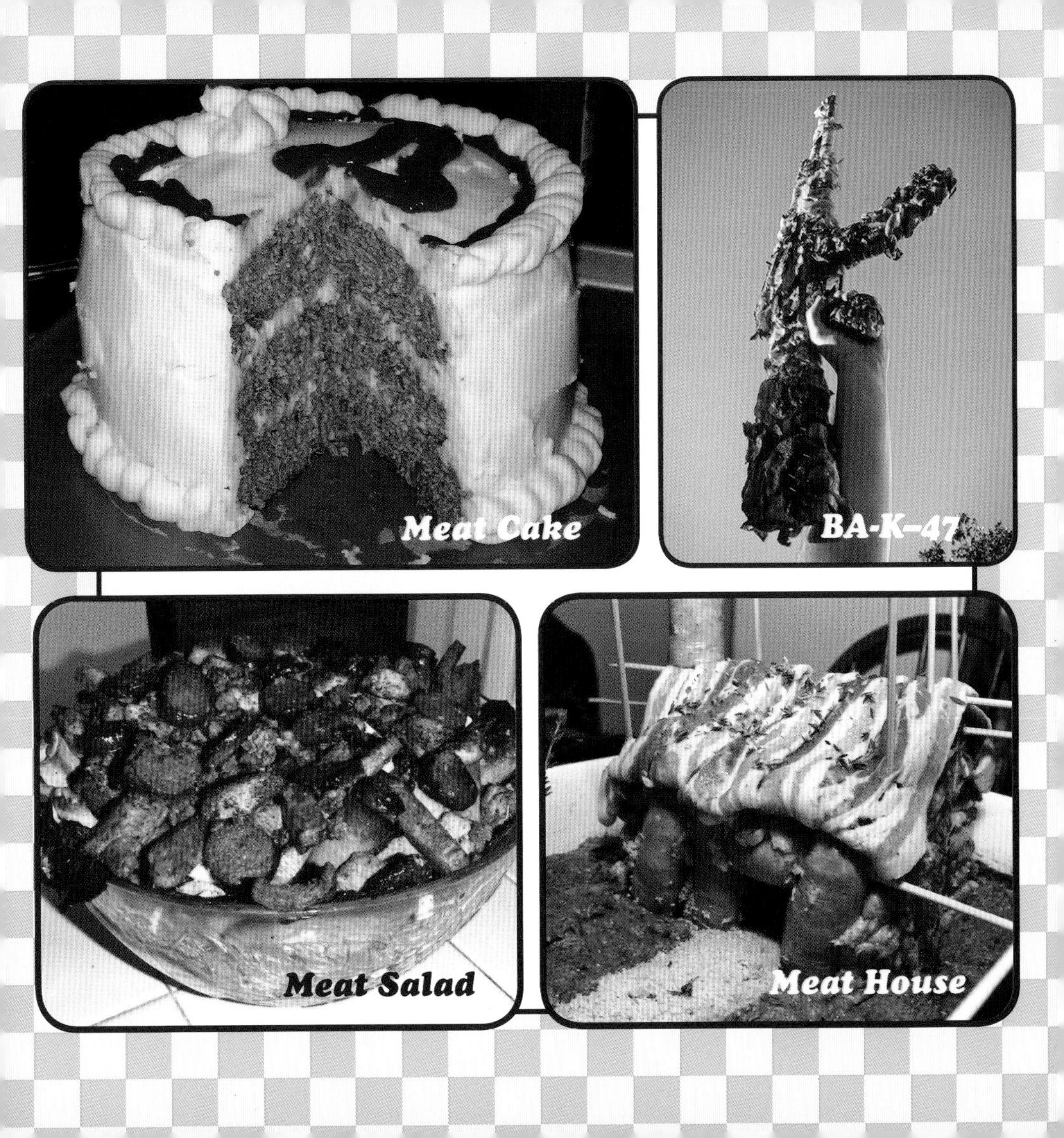
Meat Cake
BA-K-47
Meat Salad
Meat House

Fried Guac Bites

Recipe by Rick Blakeley

4 Hass avocados
2 tomatoes, chopped
1/2 large red onion, chopped
1/2 bunch fresh cilantro, chopped
3 limes' worth of fresh lime juice
4 garlic cloves, chopped
1 tsp cumin
1 tbsp paprika
1/2 cup salsa (Del Monte, Pace, your homemade or favorite)
1 package of guacamole seasoning
1/2 tsp sea salt
1/2 tsp freshly ground pepper
4 eggs
3 tbsp water
1 cup flour
1cup breadcrumbs
oil for frying

Peel and pit avocados and mash. Fold in tomatoes, onion, cilantro, lime juice, chopped garlic, cumin, paprika, salsa, guacamole seasoning, salt, and pepper. Line an 8-inch square baking pan with plastic wrap. Spoon avocado mixture into pan; spread into an even layer. Place a sheet of plastic wrap directly on the surface and freeze until solid. At least an hour before serving, beat eggs with the water in a separate bowl. Cut the avocado into small

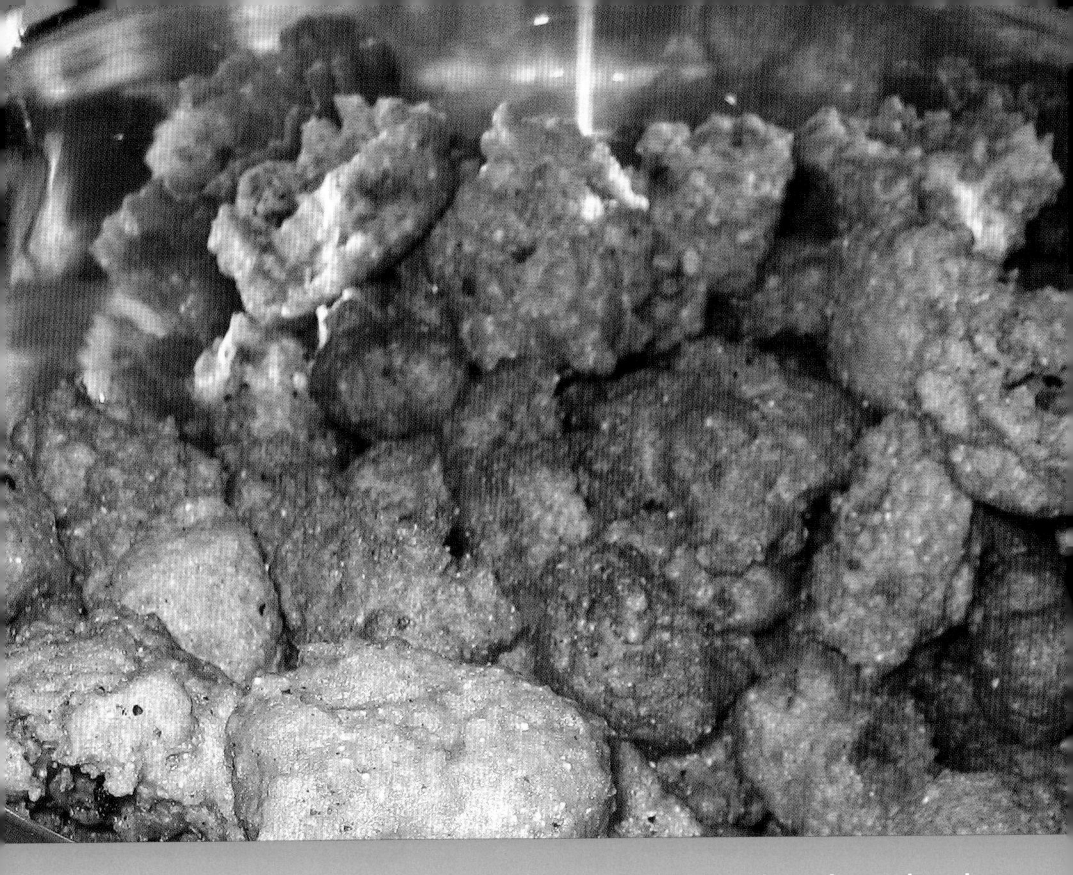

cubes. Dip each cube in flour, then the egg wash, breadcrumbs, and again in wash and breadcrumbs. Arrange in a large baking pan; cover and return to the freezer until firm (about 25 minutes). Heat oil in a pot to 350°F. Fry frozen guacamole bites in batches until golden; drain on paper towels.

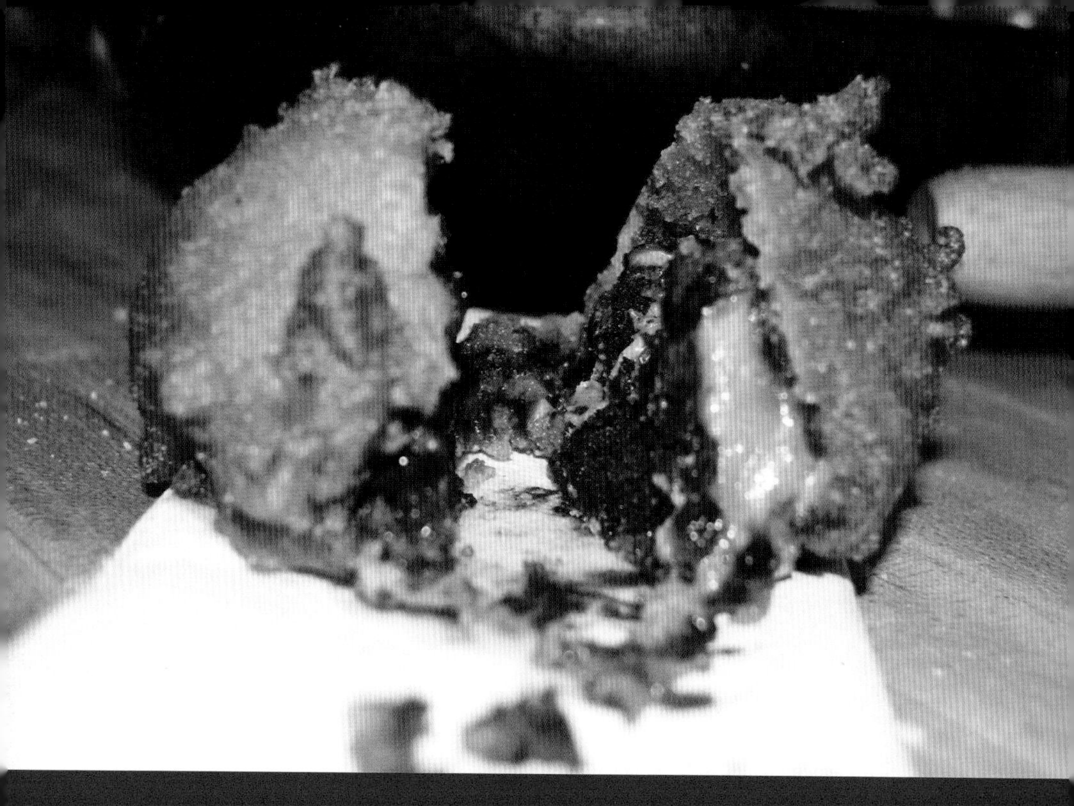

The Deep-Fried Brownie Ball

A deep-fried peanut butter-covered brownie wrapped in cookie dough.

The Kannibal

Four beef patties, one ham sausage patty, one fried egg, and sliced ham covered in minced beef, all in an oversize bun.

LOCAL FAVE!

Jaskan Grilli
Helsinki, Finland

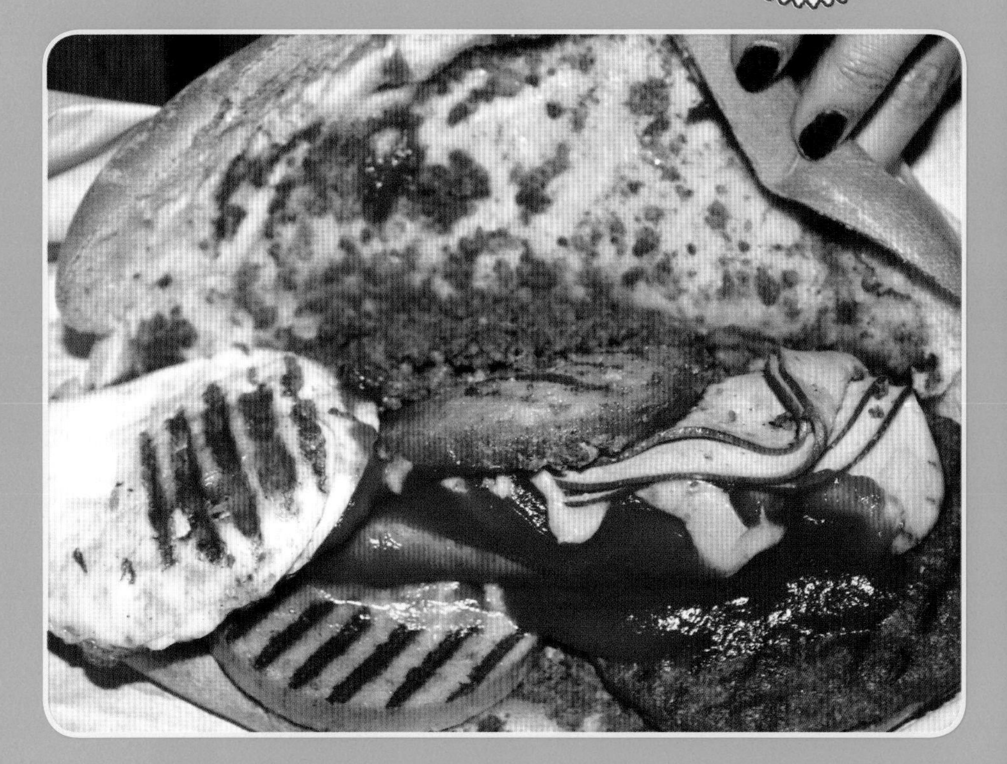

Bacon Mac and Cheese Meatloaf

Recipe by Kyle Kestell and Jameel Winter

2 lbs ground chuck, 80% lean
2 eggs
2 slices wheat bread, crumbled
2 tbsp ketchup
1 large garlic clove, minced
2 tbsp parsley, minced
Worcestershire sauce to taste
Cayenne pepper to taste
Salt to taste
Black pepper to taste
1 1/4 cups onion, sliced
10 strips of bacon
Premade macaroni and cheese

Mix ground chuck, eggs, bread, ketchup, garlic, parsley, Worcestershire sauce, cayenne pepper, salt, and black pepper with hands in a large bowl. Meanwhile, sweat onion until translucent but not brown. Allow onions to cool, then add to meat mixture. Cover bowl with plastic wrap and move to refrigerator. Preheat oven to 375°F. Lay bacon across the width of a loaf pan. Press a layer of meat into the bottom of the pan, on top of the bacon. This layer should fill exactly one third of the loaf pan. Scoop some of the macaroni and cheese into the loaf pan, making sure to press out any air bubbles. This layer

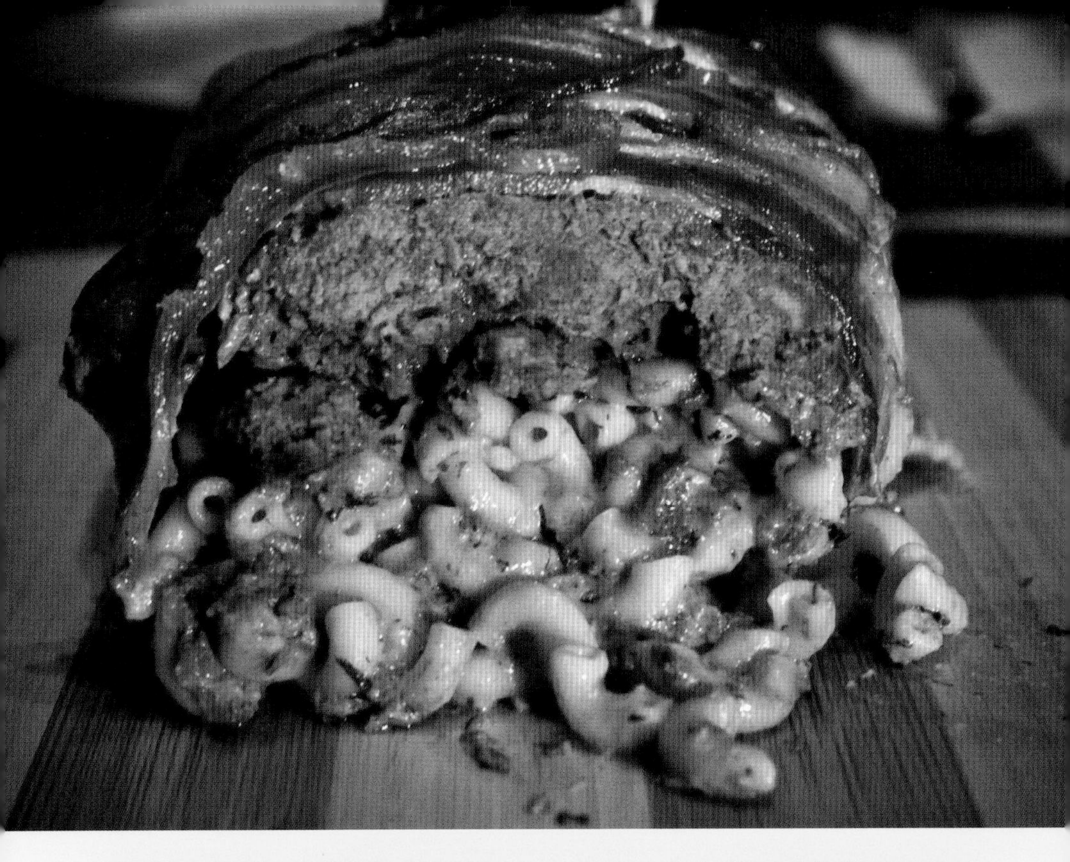

should also fill one third of the loaf pan. Form a slab of meat in the approximate size and shape of the remaining one third of the loaf pan. Transfer the slab to the loaf pan. Add or remove meat as necessary to ensure a snug fit. Fold strips of bacon back over the top of the meatloaf. Roast until internal temperature reaches 160°F.

White Castle Casserole

Recipe by Mr. Dave

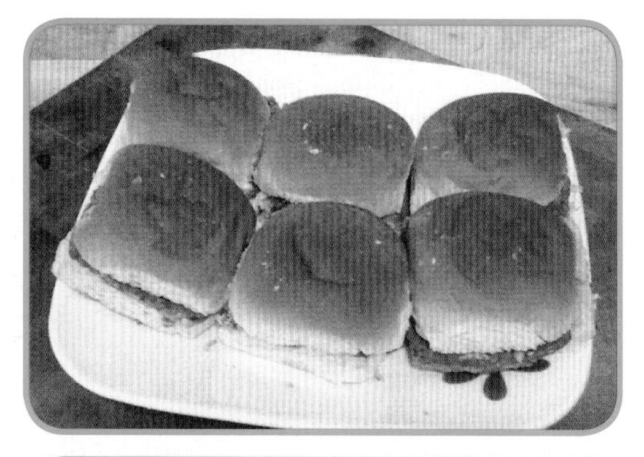

Remove the tops from White Castle Burgers and arrange them compactly in an oven-proof dish. Layer cheese and strips of bacon on top of sliders. Whisk together 1 cup milk and 4 eggs seasoned with salt and pepper. Pour egg mixture over the sliders, making sure as much liquid as possible is absorbed. Replace tops and let the sliders soak for about 30 minutes and then top with more cheese. Bake at 350°F for about 45 minutes.

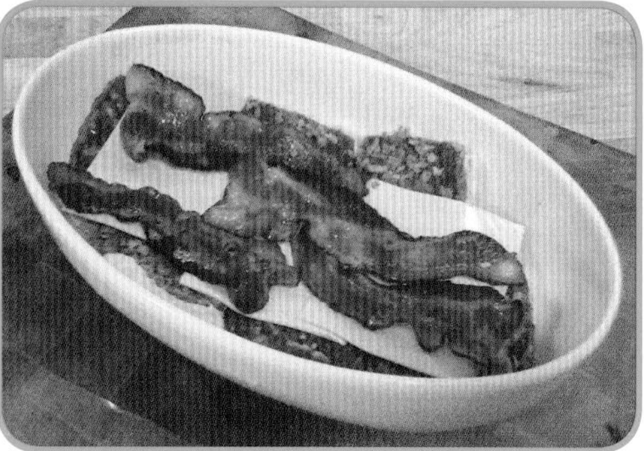

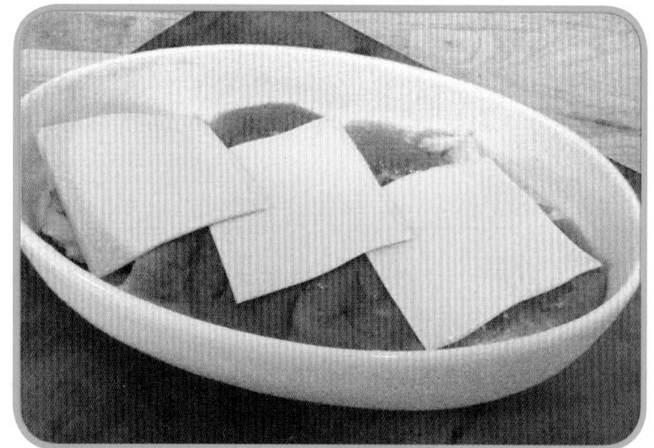

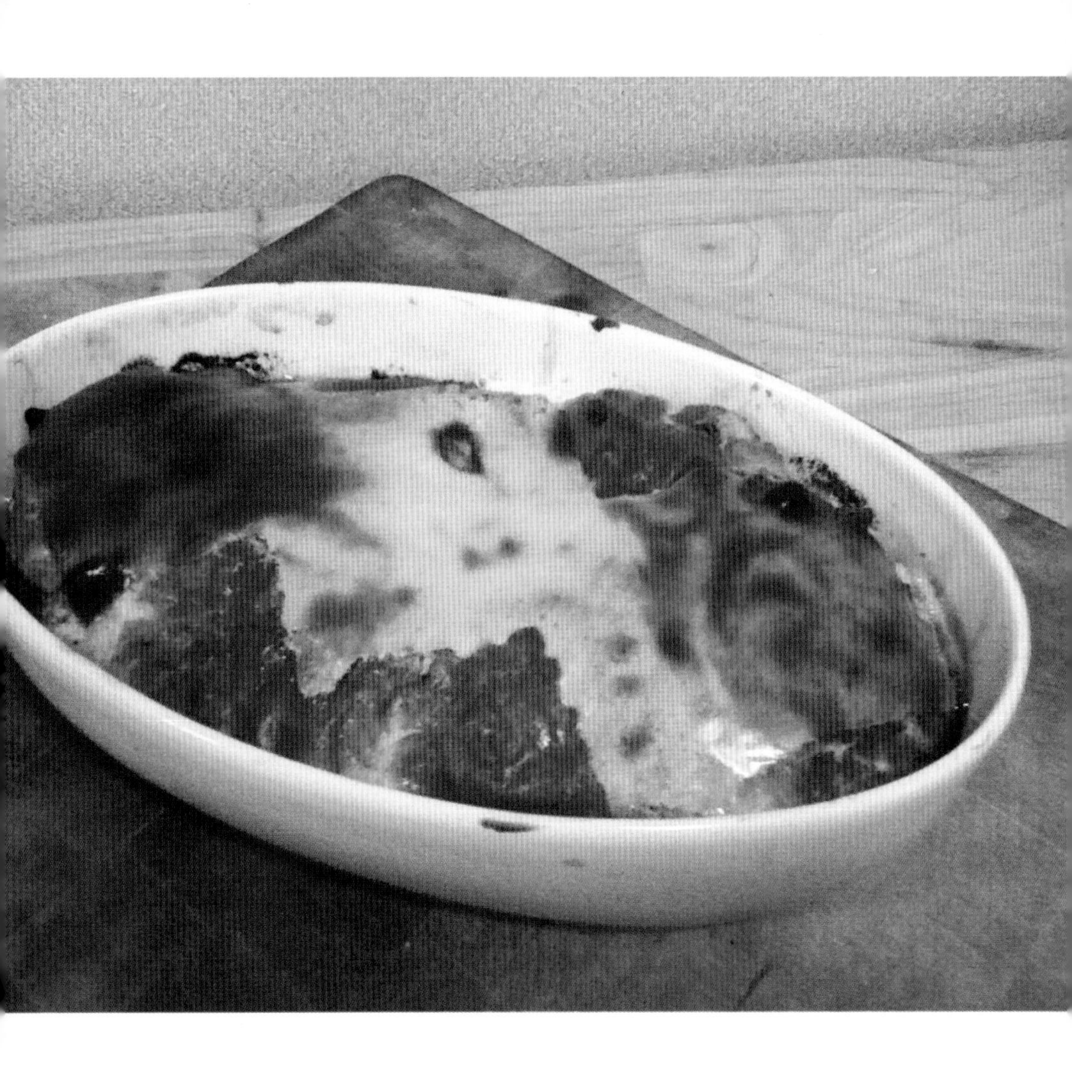

Cake Out!

What's better than cake? The answer is not much else. Unless, of course, we're talking about cakes that look like other delicious foods. Cakes so realistic and tempting, your brain will hurt almost as much as your stomach in its attempt to digest the culinary trick we like to call a "cake out."

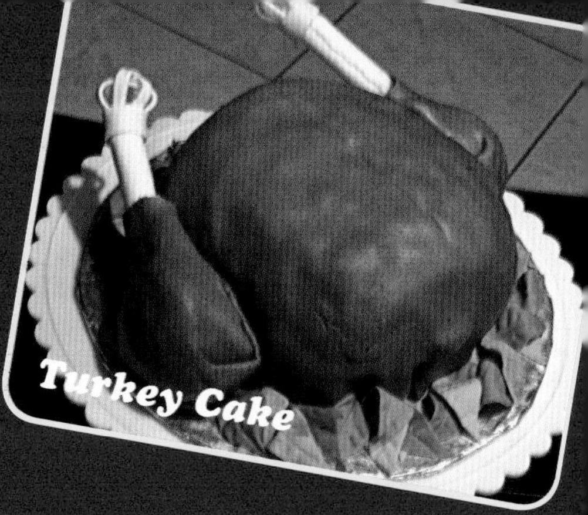

Turkey Cake

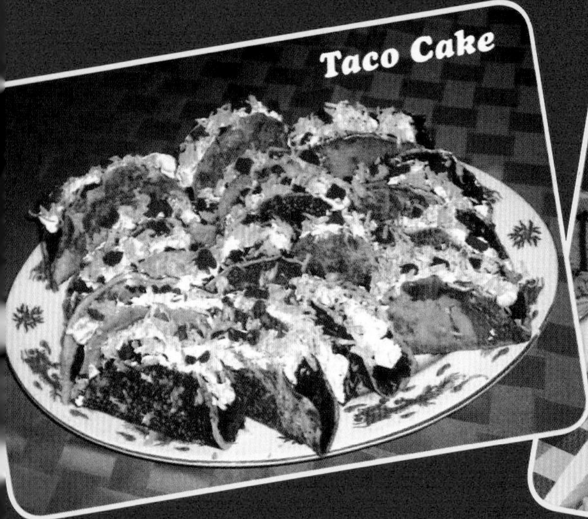

Taco Cake

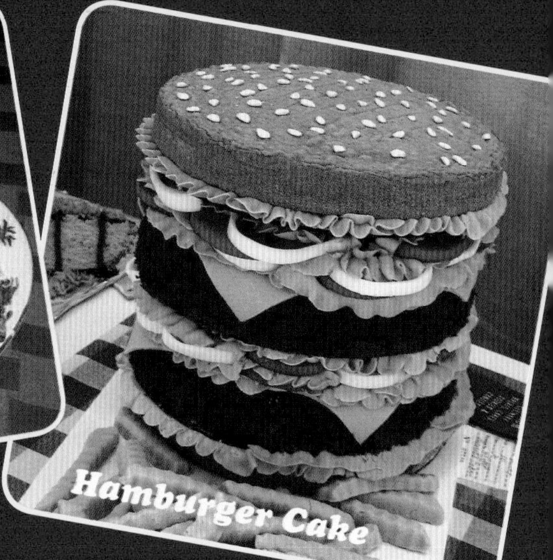

Hamburger Cake

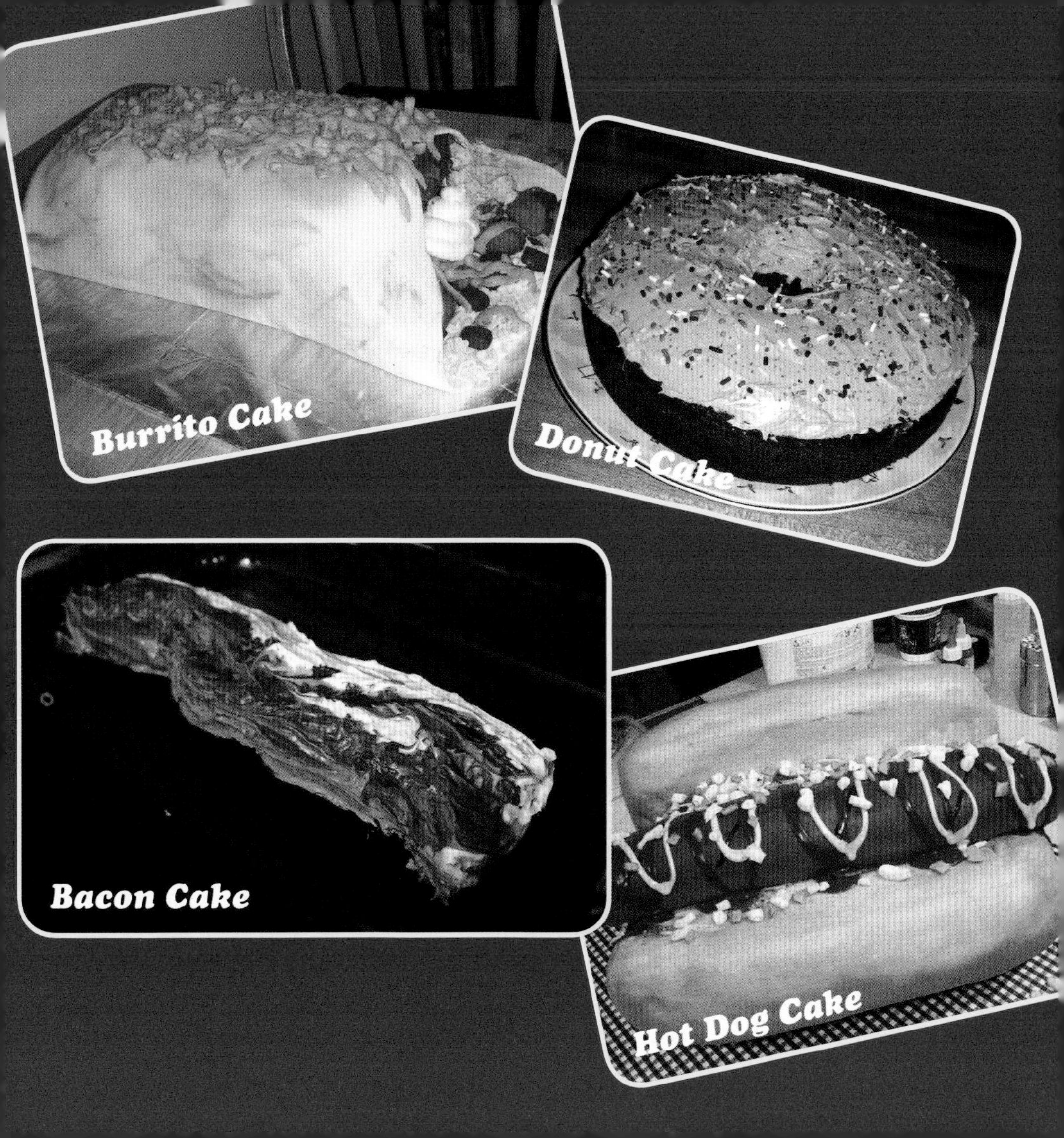
Burrito Cake
Donut Cake
Bacon Cake
Hot Dog Cake

Deep-Fried Coke

Recipe by Stephen Witherden

2 cups flour
1 tsp baking powder
2 eggs
1 $^{1}/_{2}$ cups Coke
Whipped cream
Maraschino cherries

Mix together flour and baking powder. Add eggs and Coke and mix until a batter is formed. Pour $^{1}/_{3}$ cup batter into a funnel, dropper, or turkey baster and pour into a skillet filled with oil. Fry for a minute on each side.

Serve warm, garnished with whipped cream and a maraschino cherry.

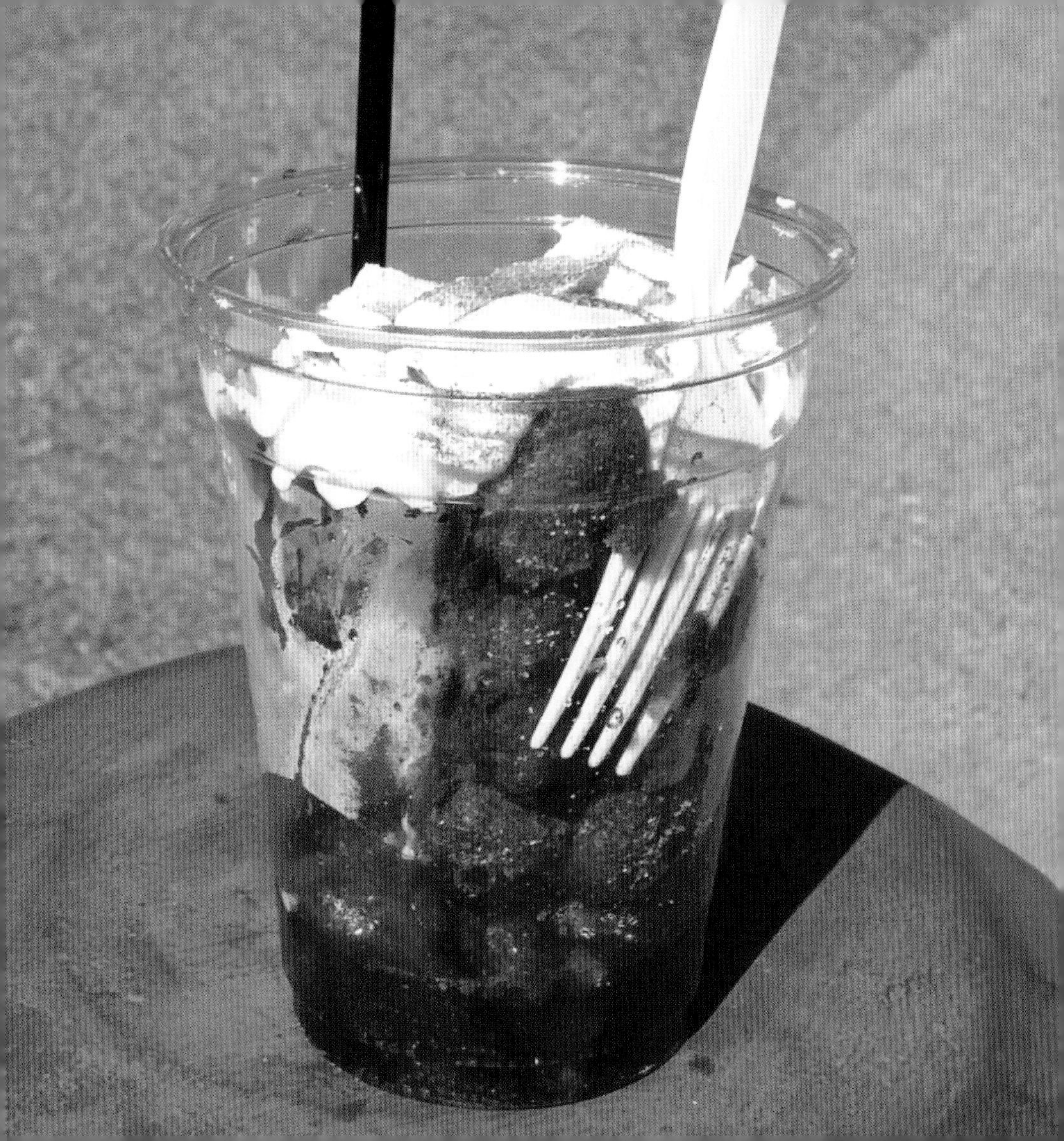

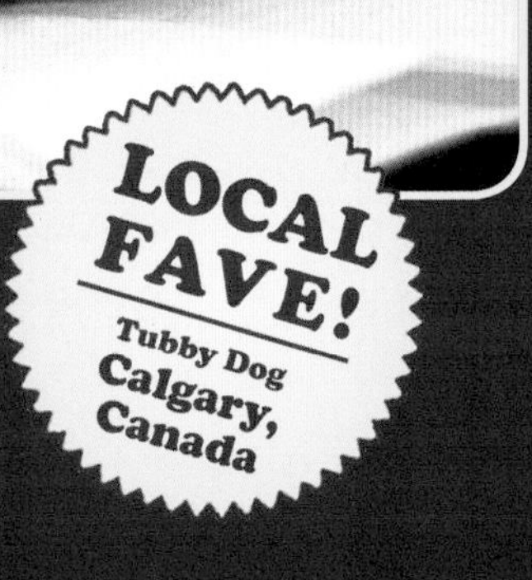

Tubby Dog

A hot dog topped with chili, bacon, cheese, onions, and mustard.

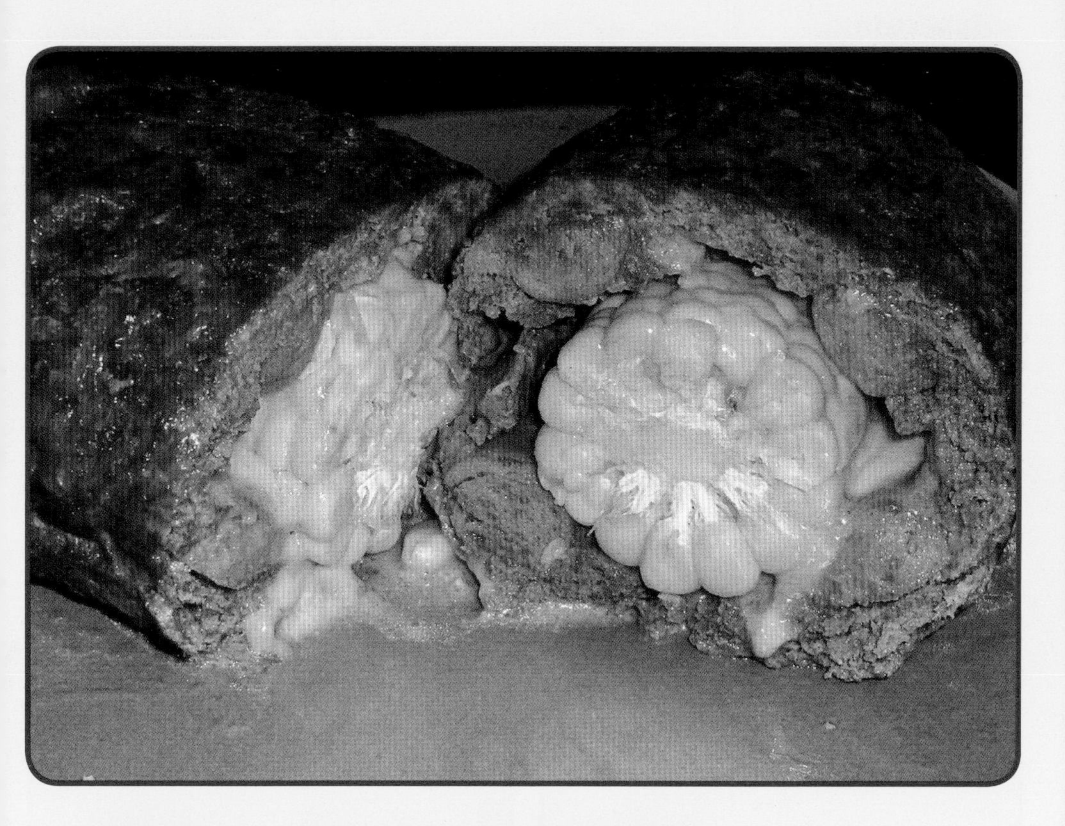

The Cornhole

Corn on the cob wrapped in hickory bacon with two hot dogs and two Colby-Jack cheese sticks all wrapped in ground beef.

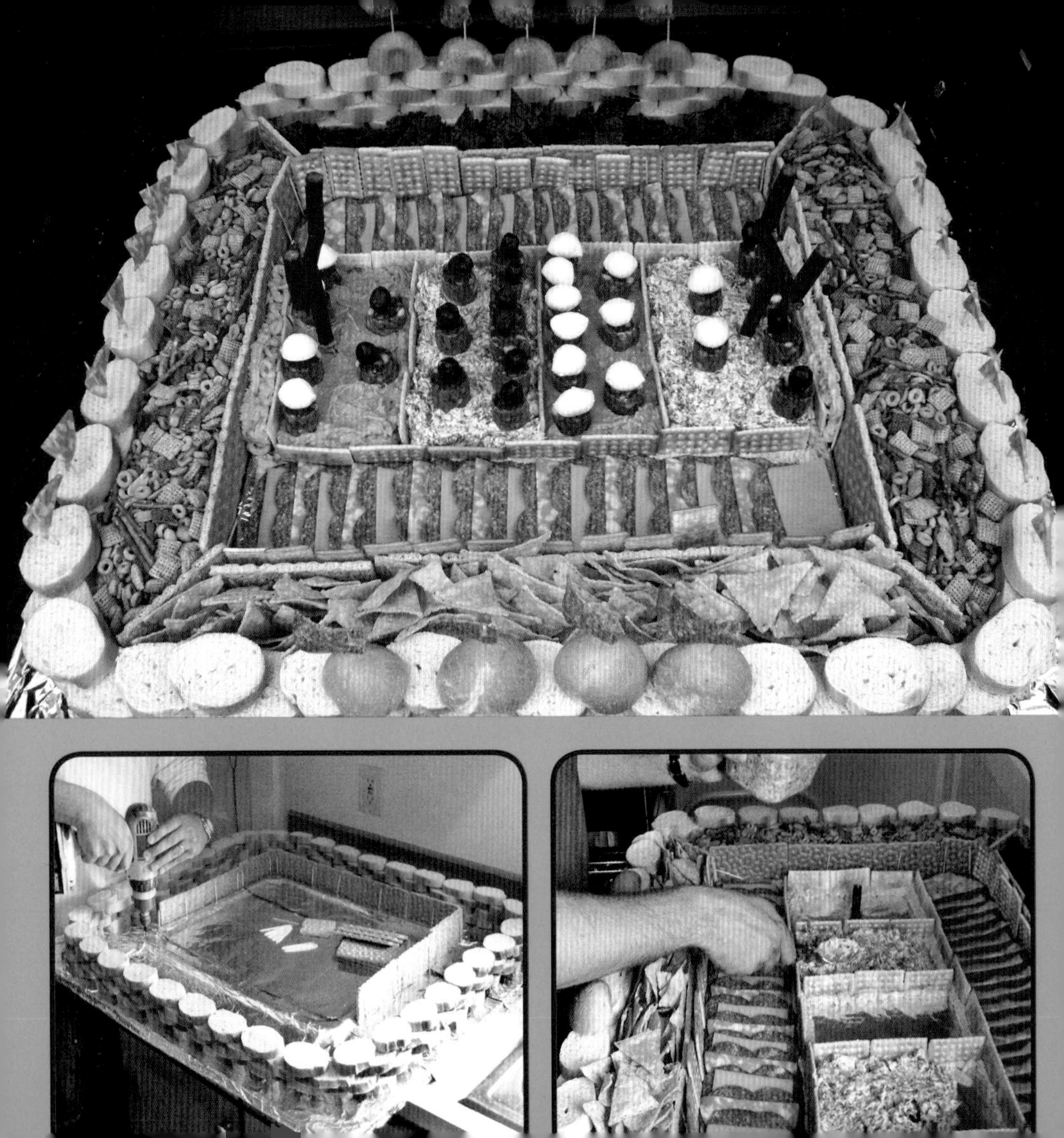

Snack Stadium

Recipe by Nate and Dave

5 loaves of bread for the stadium walls
2 kinds of tortilla chips to surround walls
2 kinds of crackers and Easy Cheese for borders
Guacamole for field
Spinach dip for field
Pepperoni sticks for walls and field lines
Homemade Chex mix for walls
Sausages and cheese for sidelines
Hungarian sausage used for the players' bodies
Black olives for team one's helmets
White mini mozzarella balls for team two's helmets
Tillamook Beef Sticks for goal posts
2 aluminum pans
Lots and lots of toothpicks

14-Pie Pie

Recipe by Ben McLeod, Alex Chan, George Organ, Allan McGregor, John Psegianakis, Joel Roncevich, and Peter Schmidt

3 sheets shortcrust pastry
1/4 cup carrots, diced
1/4 cup potatoes, diced
2 garlic cloves, diced
4 cups gravy
3 sheets puff pastry
1 egg, beaten

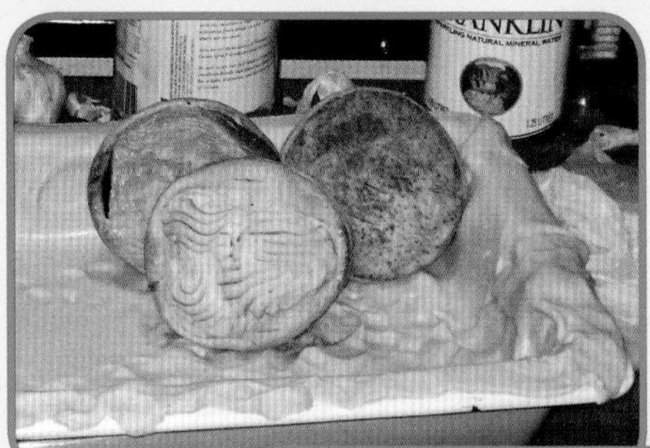

14 PIES:

- Chunky beef
- Beef, bacon, and cheese
- Beef bolognese
- Beef and potato
- Beef and red chilli beans
- Beef, tomato, and onion
- Lamb, rosemary, and Shiraz
- Steak, mushroom, and Guinness
- Chicken, leek, and corn

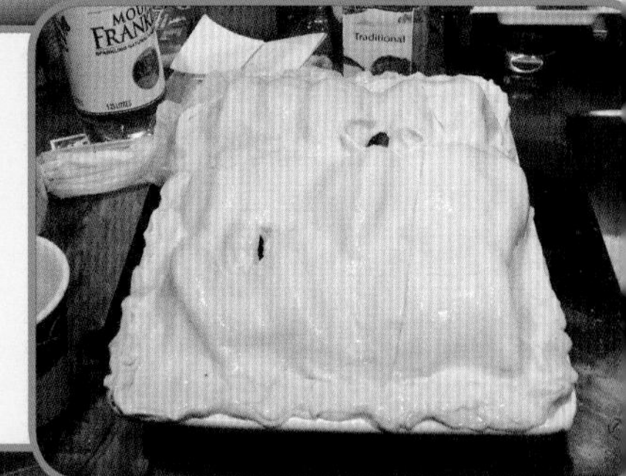

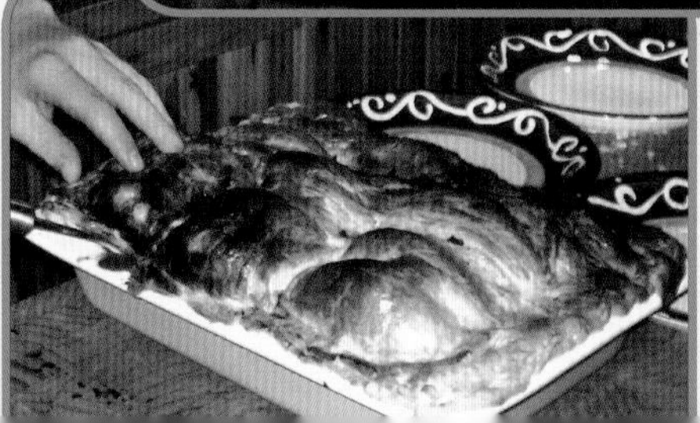

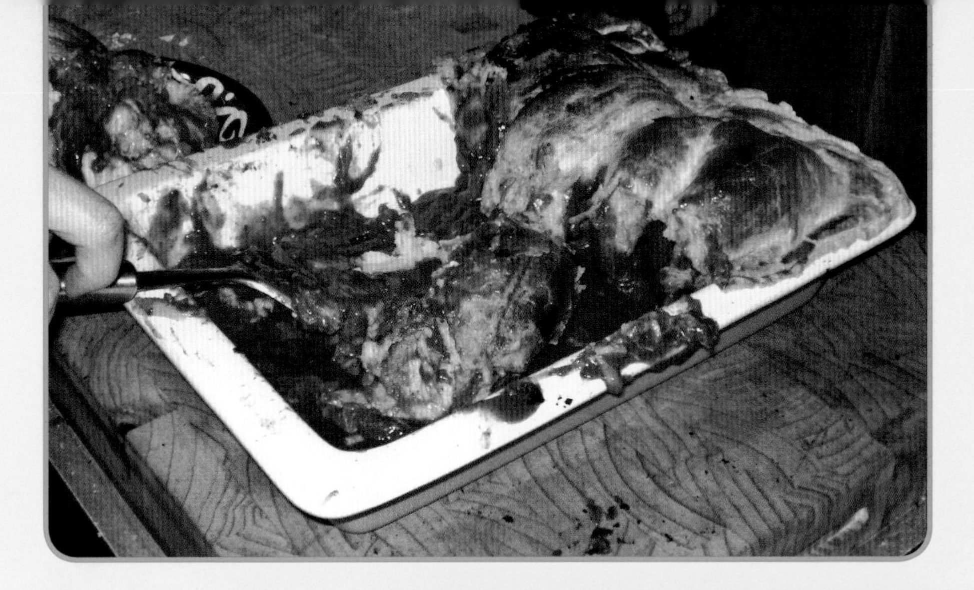

- Moroccan chicken
- Tandoori chicken
- Chickpea and curried vegetable with eggplant and coconut-milk sauce
- Dhansak and curried vegetables
- Tomato, coriander, and lentil

Line a large greased oven dish with shortcrust pastry. Preheat oven to 350°F and prebake for about 10 minutes. Set aside to cool. In a medium saucepan, sauté the carrots, potatoes, and garlic in olive oil or butter until soft. Add the gravy and simmer on low heat for 10 minutes. Line up the pies inside the dish, standing them on their sides. Add enough gravy to the dish so it comes to roughly ½ inch below the top of the dish. Cover with a layer of puff pastry. Brush pastry with the beaten egg. Bake at 350°F for about 45 minutes, or until the pastry is golden brown.

Frito Pie

Recipe by Mona Meline

1 snack-size bag Fritos corn chips
1 can chili
Shredded cheddar cheese
Sour cream
Diced onion
Green chili peppers
Jalapeños

With scissors, cut an opening in the middle of the Fritos bag and pull back to expose corn chips. Pour heated chili over corn chips. Add a generous helping of cheddar cheese. Top with sour cream, diced onion, green chili peppers, and jalapeños.

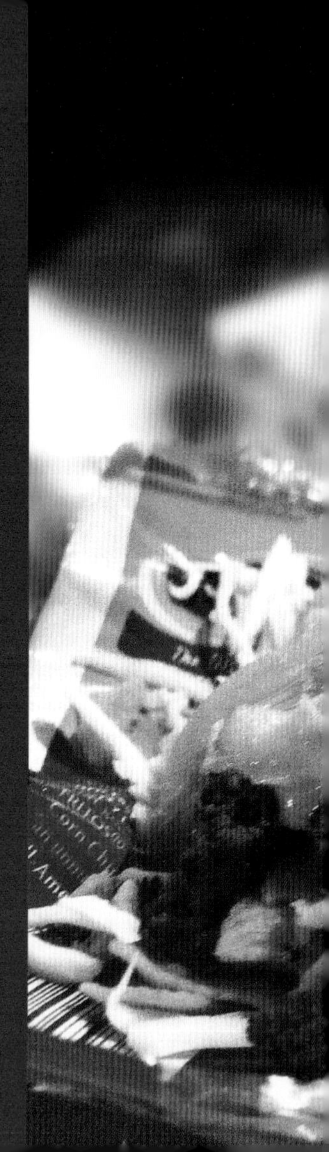

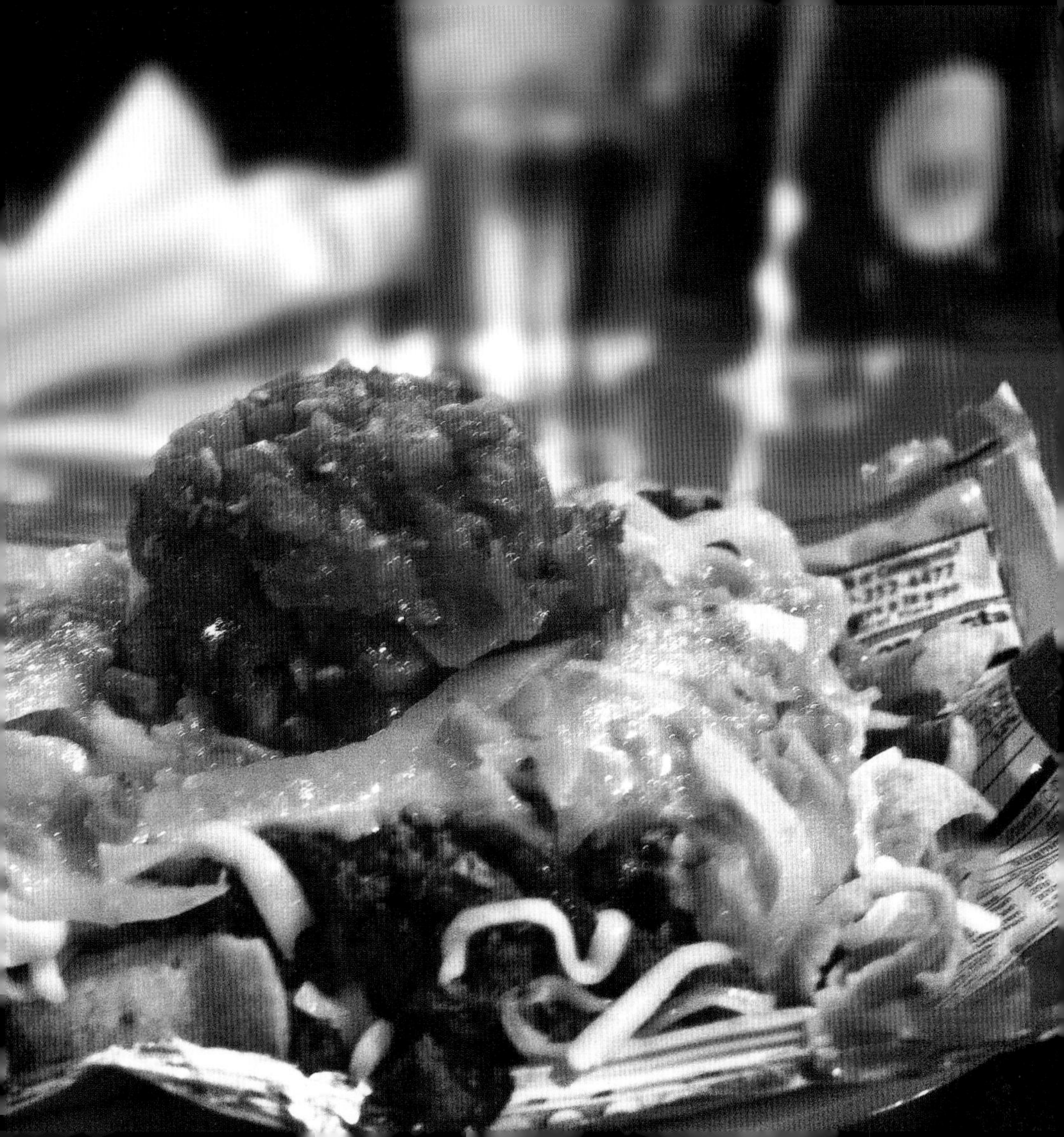

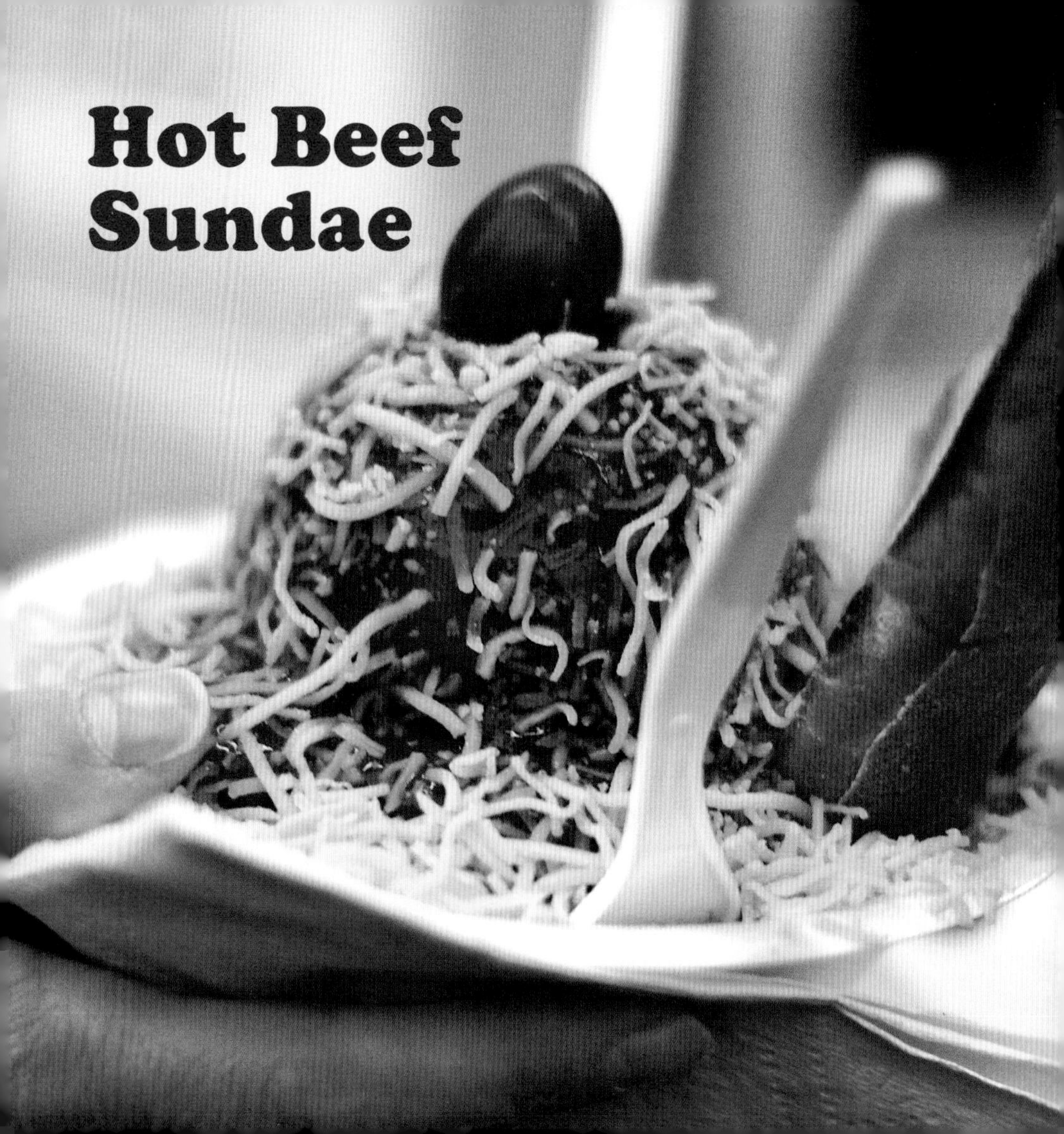

Hot Beef Sundae

Breakfasts of Champions

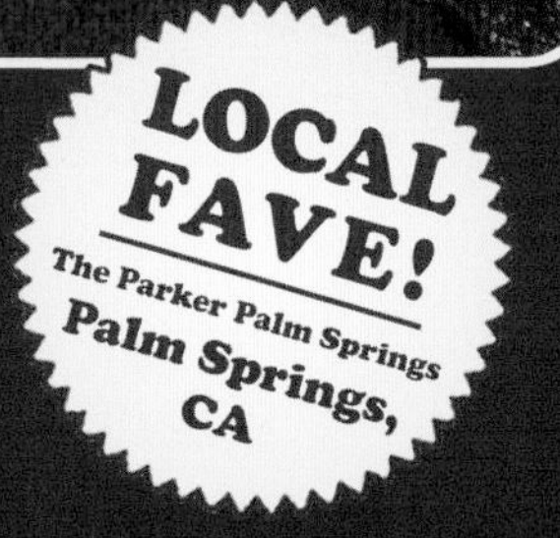

Cheesy French Toast

Three slices of egg-battered brioche, filled and slathered with melted cheese.

Elvis Donut

Peanut butter–glazed donut topped with bananas and bacon.

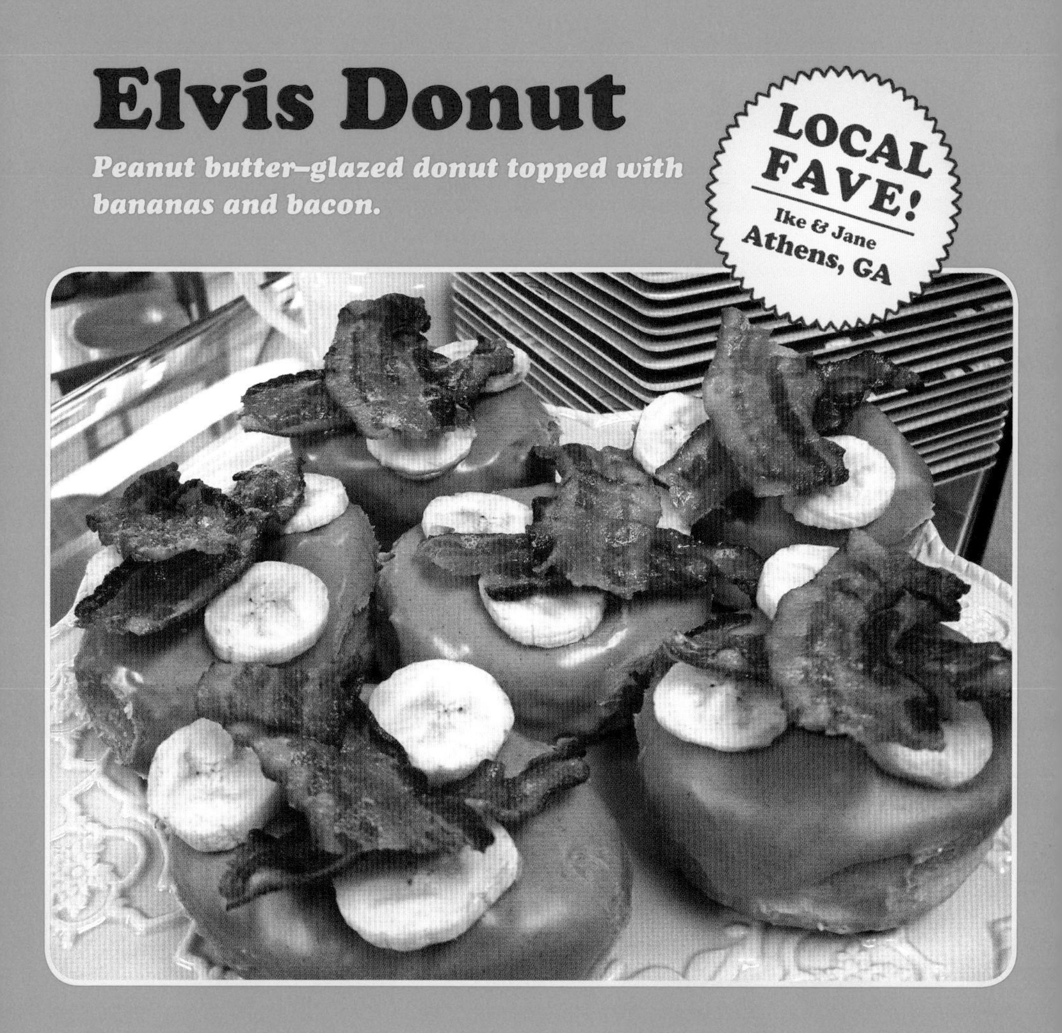

Bacon Cinnamon Rolls

Recipe by Andy Phelan

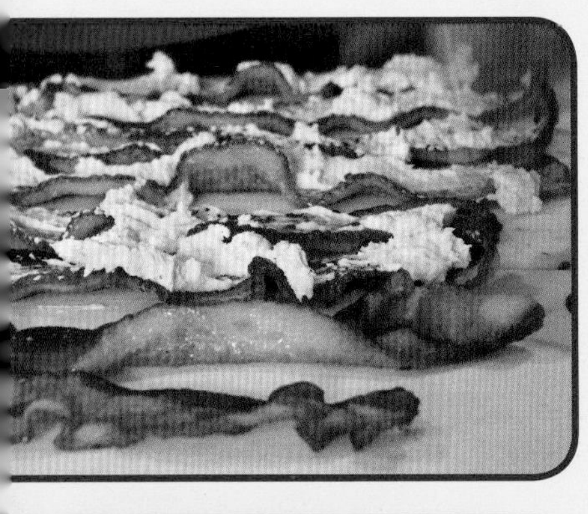

1 container bacon strips
1 container cream cheese
1 roll ready-to-cook
cinnamon rolls

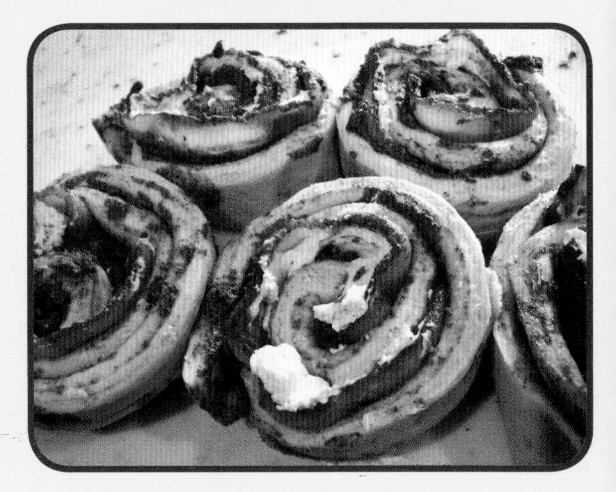

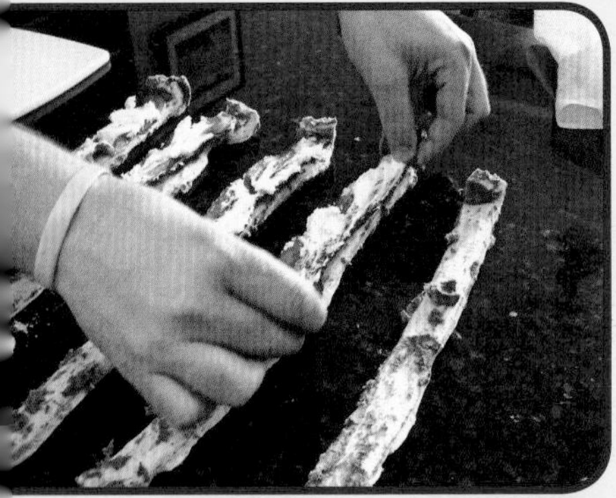

Cook the bacon in a pan until one side is mostly done—but not fully cooked through. Dry the bacon of grease, then slather the mostly cooked side of the bacon with cream cheese. Unroll the cinnamon rolls on a hard surface. Place the cream cheese–slathered bacon onto the unrolled cinnamon rolls. Roll the cinnamon rolls back up with the cream cheese bacon inside. Place the rolls on a nonstick baking sheet and bake for 17 to 20 minutes at 350°F. Remove from oven and top with icing provided in the cinnamon roll packaging.

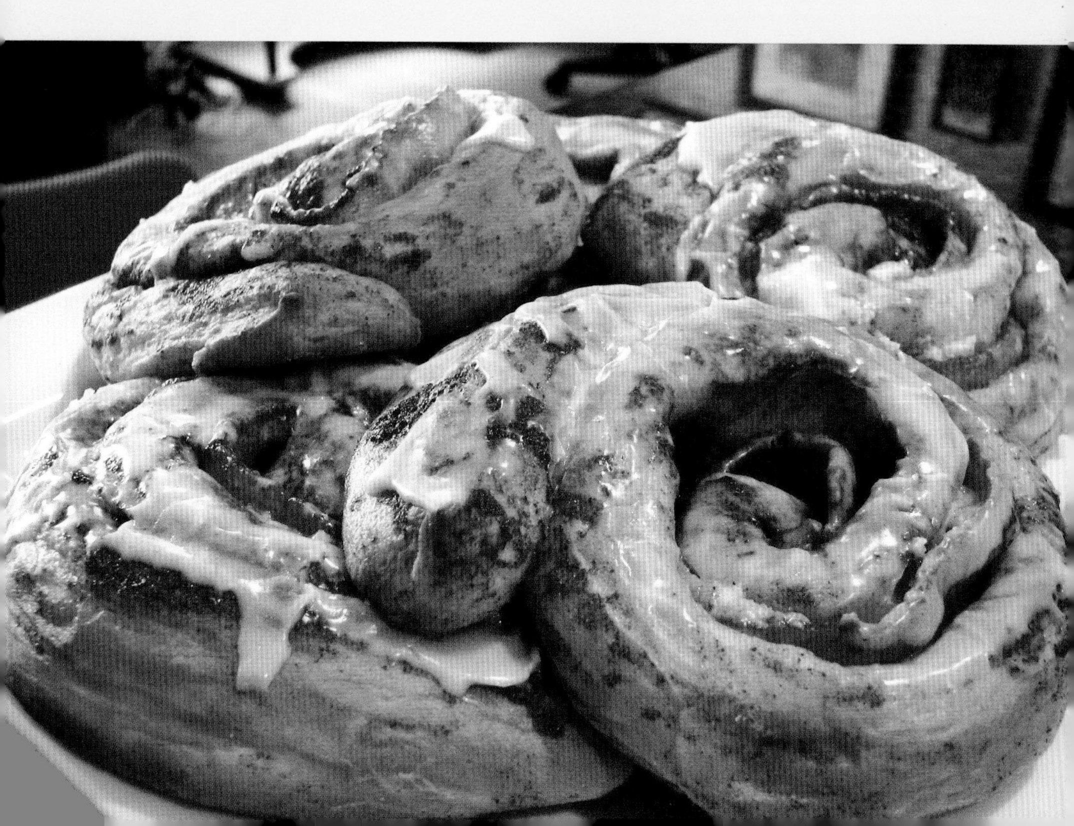

Country Breakfast Parfait

Sausage gravy, chicken-fried steak bites, Tater Tots, and buttermilk biscuit chunks layered together in a pint glass, topped with a fried egg and bacon.

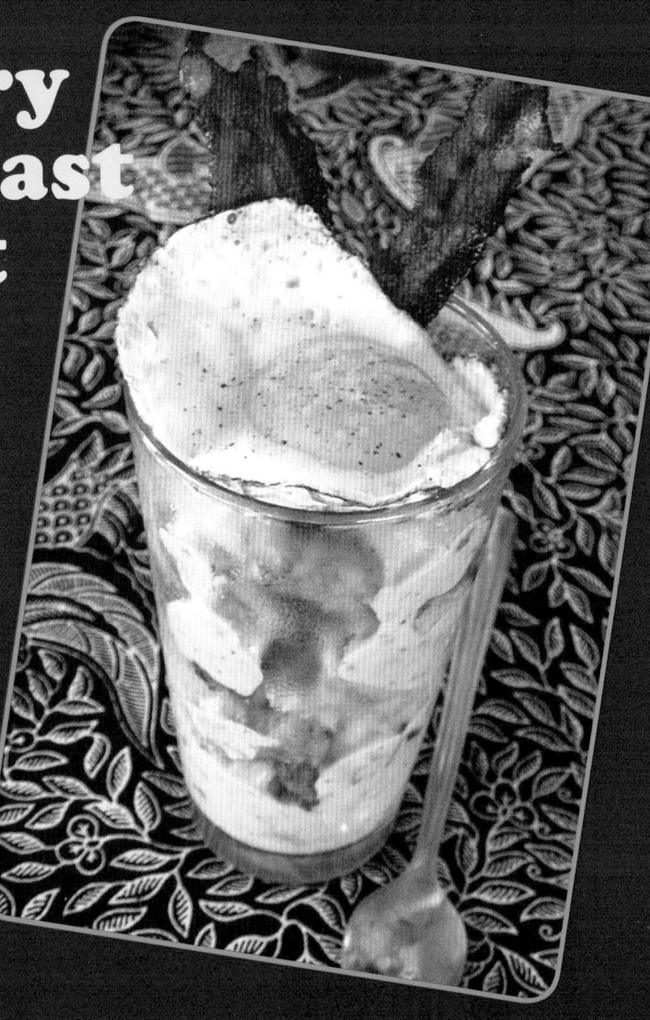

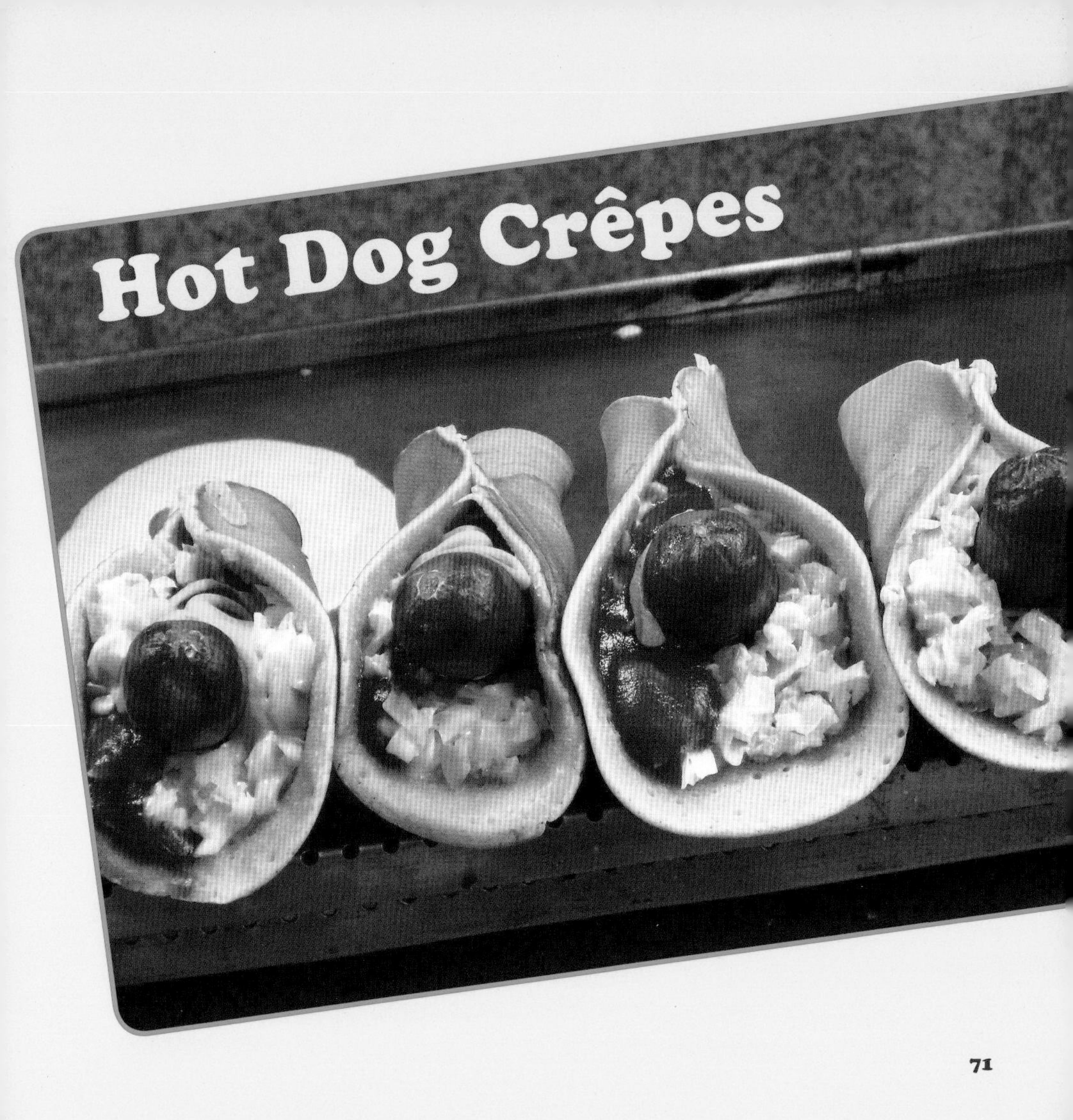
Hot Dog Crêpes

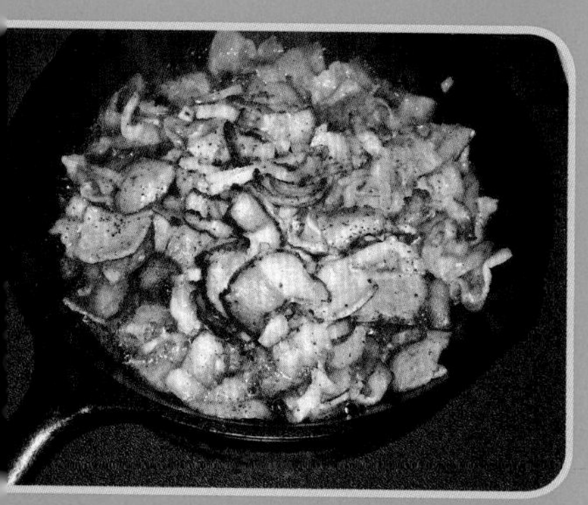

Breakfast Fatty

Recipe by Thomas Lester

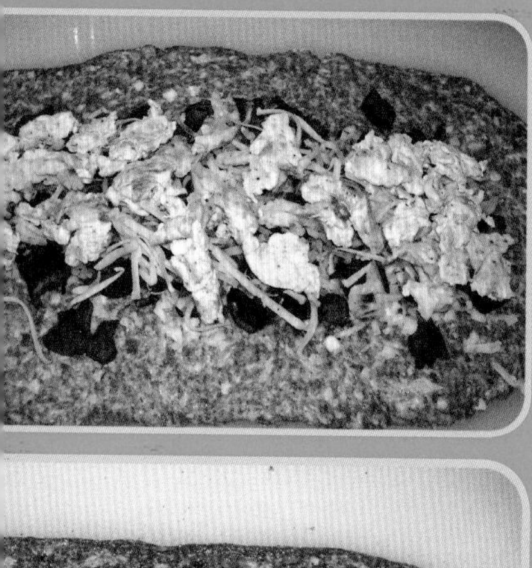

1 lb Jimmy Dean sausage
1 pancake
Maple syrup
3 eggs, scrambled
Shredded cheddar cheese
6 bacon strips (approximately)
3 bacon strips, cut up

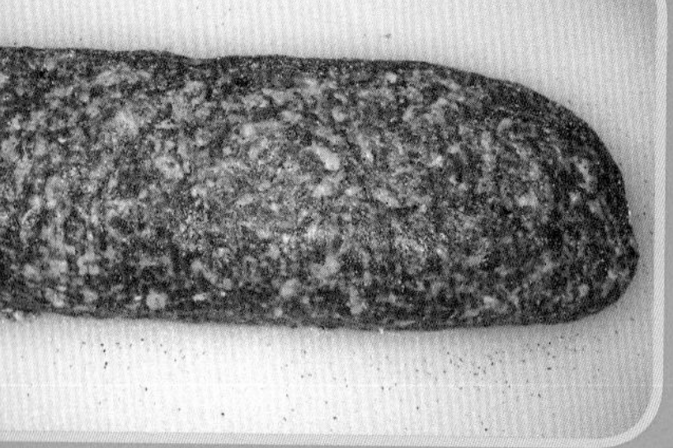

Roll out 1 pound of Jimmy Dean sausage as flat as you can. Rip up the pancake and put it on the rolled-out sausage. Drizzle the pancake with maple syrup. Spread the scrambled eggs over the sausage, along with a layer of shredded cheddar and cut-up pieces of bacon. Then, roll the whole thing up into a "tube" and seal the ends. Wrap the Fatty with the remaining strips of bacon to keep it from unraveling. Once all of that is done, smoke it for about 1½ hours, until the internal temperature hits 160°F.

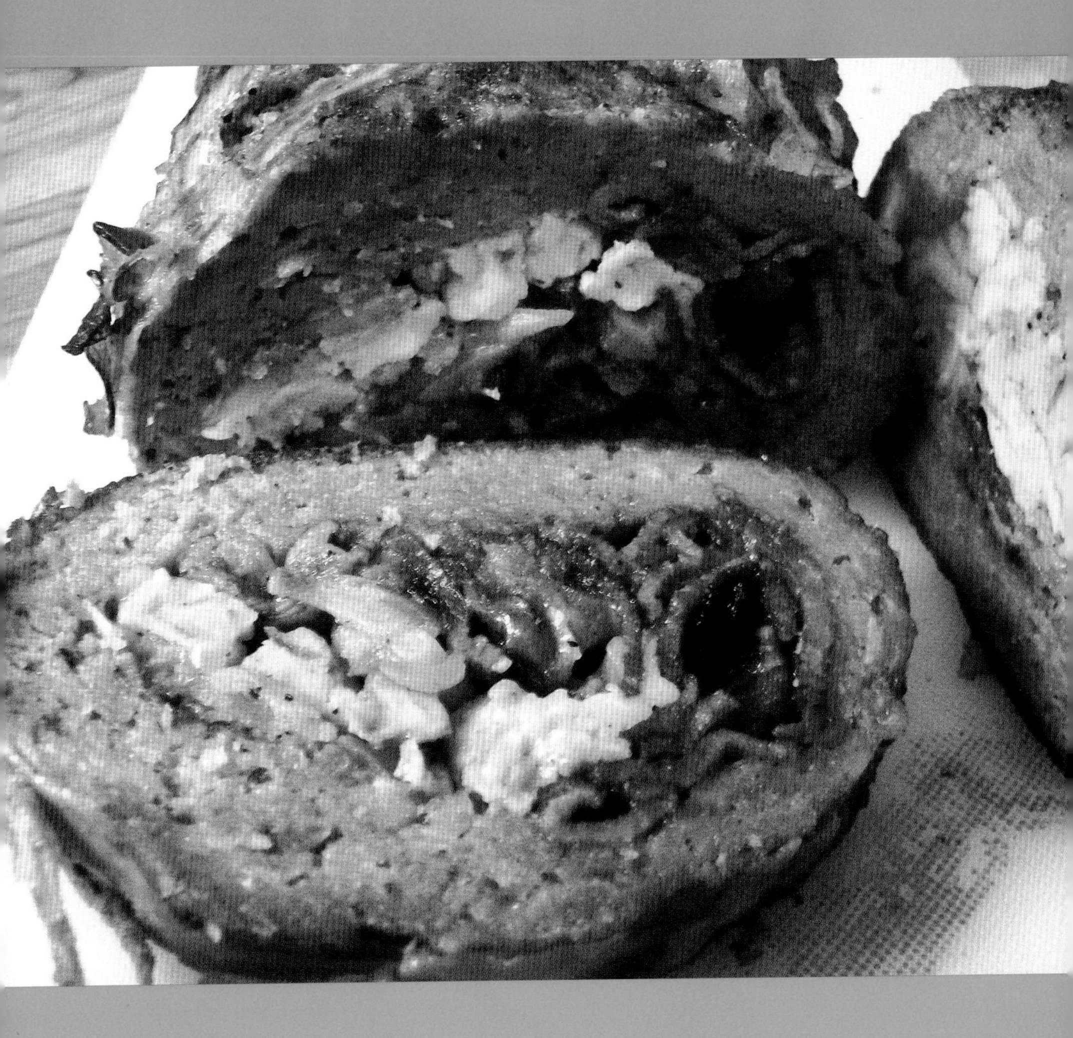

Beth's 12-Egg Omelette

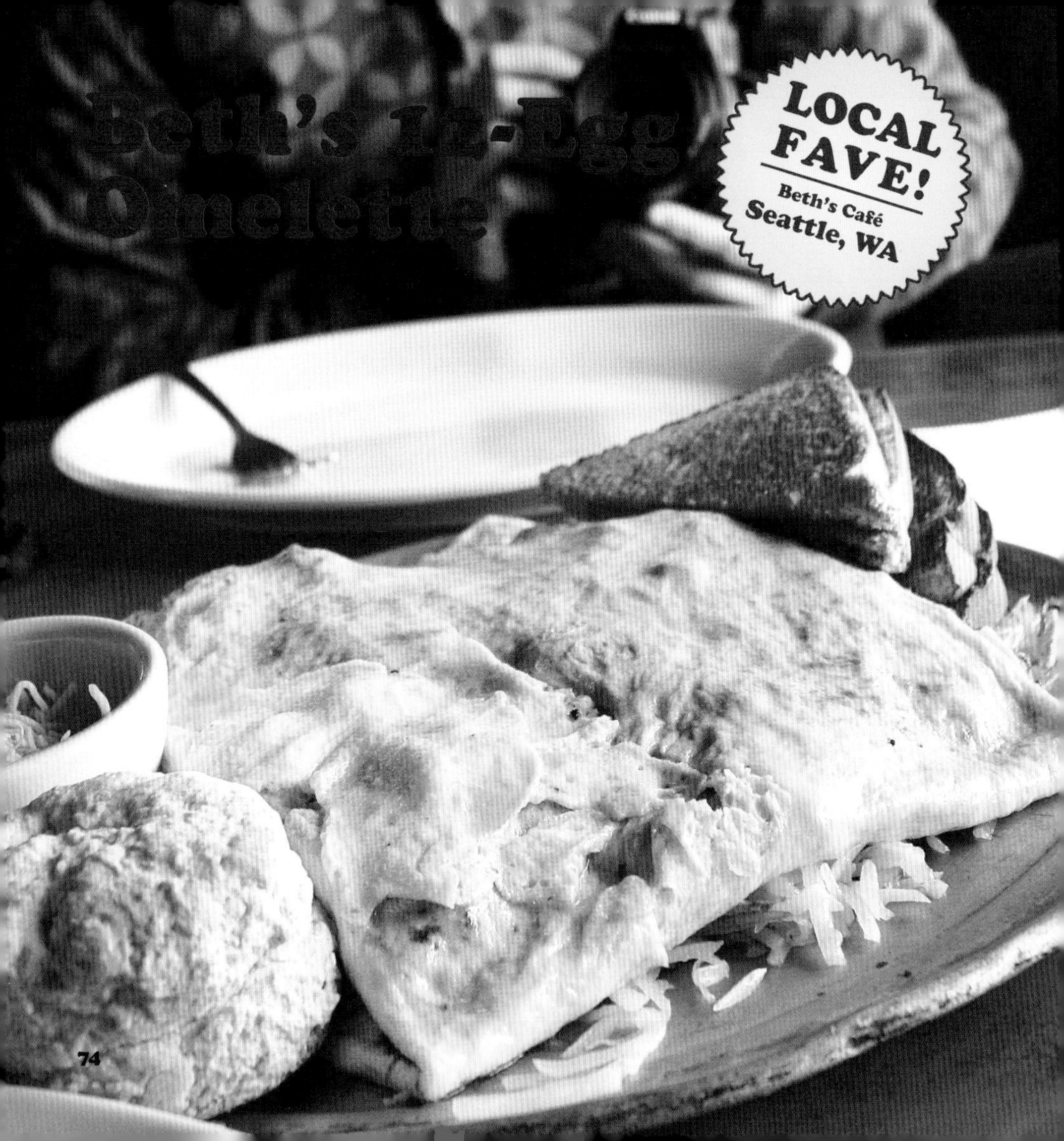

The Slinger

Hash browns covered with grilled onions with two side-by-side cheeseburgers, topped with a couple eggs fried sunny-side up, and then covered with chili and garnished with two pieces of toast.

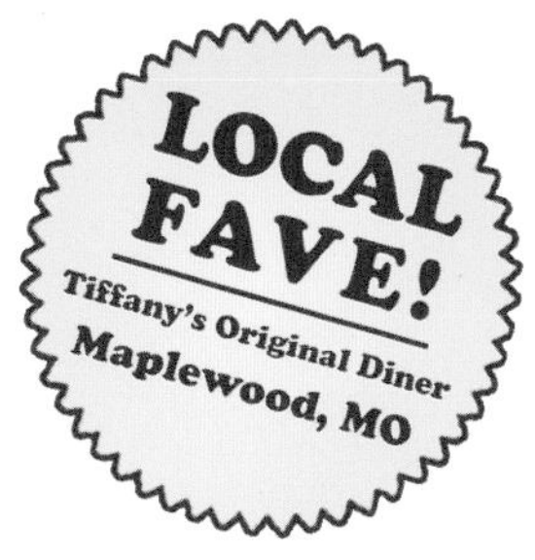

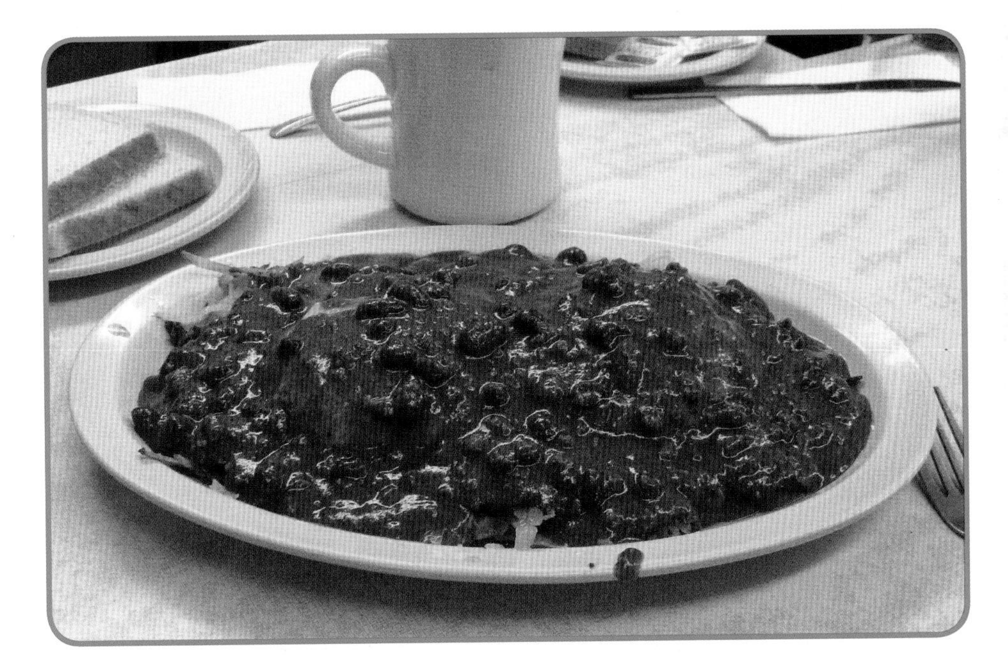

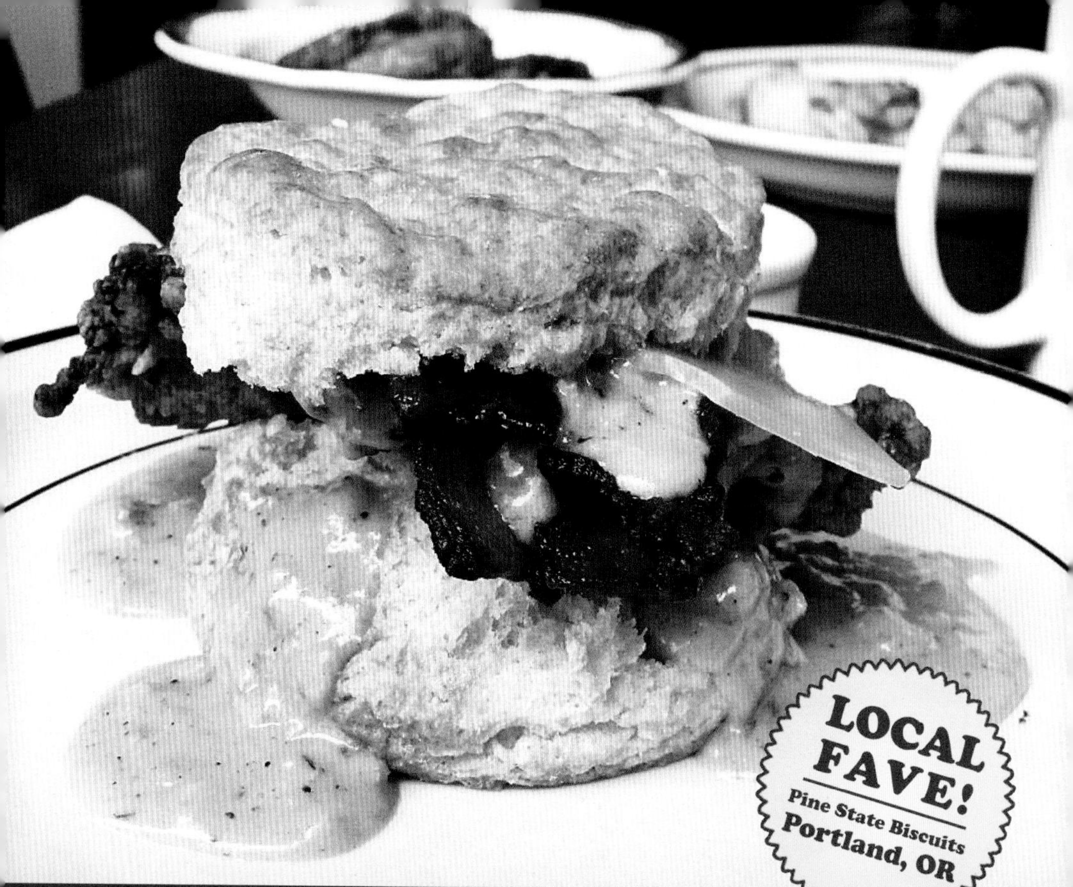

LOCAL FAVE!
Pine State Biscuits
Portland, OR

The Reggie Deluxe

Fried chicken, gravy, cheese, and bacon in a biscuit.

Country Pancake Wrap

LOCAL FAVE!
Brownstone Diner & Pancake Factory
Jersey City, NJ

Scrambled eggs, potatoes, American cheese, and bacon or sausage rolled into an oversize pancake.

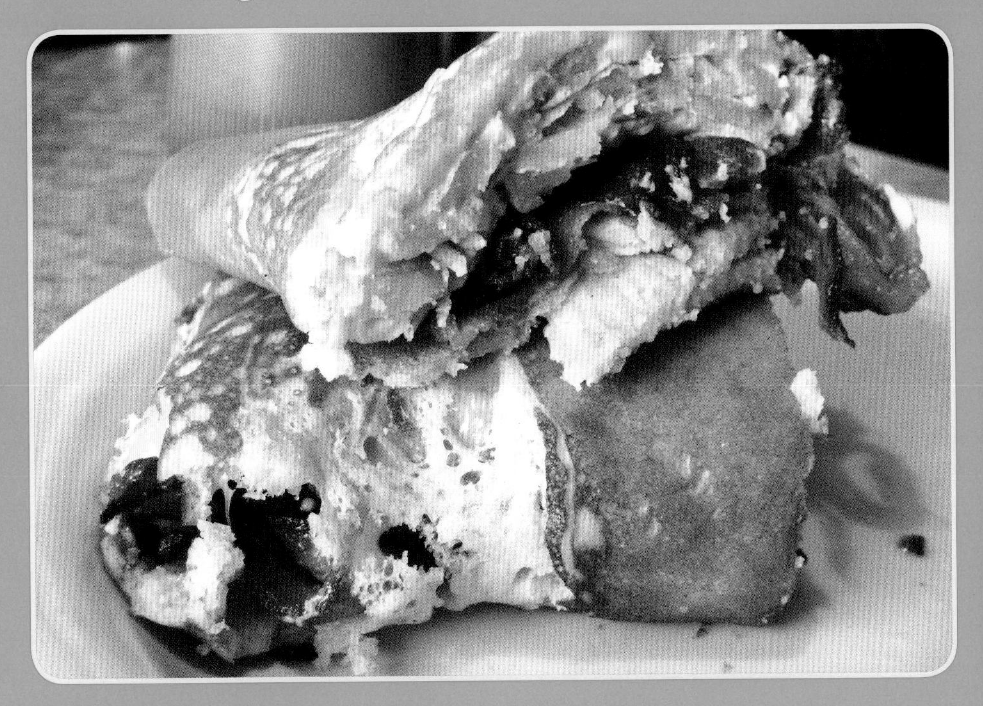

Bacon Gone Wild

The Bacone

Recipe by Christian Williams and Melissa Tillman

2 bacon strips
Eggs, scrambled
Hash browns
Colby-Jack Cheese
Country gravy
Biscuits

Roll bacon strips into shape with corresponding cone-shaped cut-outs and staple closed, wrap in aluminum foil, and fry. Ensure that the bacon is as tight against the form as possible. Fry at 400°F until solidified. After frying, remove the staples from the bacone and remove the bacone from the outer form and allow to dry for a bit. Fill the bacone with a mixture of scrambled eggs, hash browns, and cheese until almost full, and add a layer of country gravy. Top with a biscuit.

The Dawn of the Bacone

BY CHRISTIAN WILLIAMS (CREATOR OF THE BACONE)

"This is what not to do," I said to Melissa one night while pointing at the bacon cheeseburger on our local diner's menu. I was explaining the concept of San Francisco's upcoming Bacon Camp, a bacon-themed competition, which I'd just learned about and was thinking of attending. If we were going to enter anything into this celebration of all things bacon, I was adamant that our creation be something that puts bacon first. A few minutes later, I had the idea of a cone made of bacon that you hold in your hand. We laughed about filling it with a

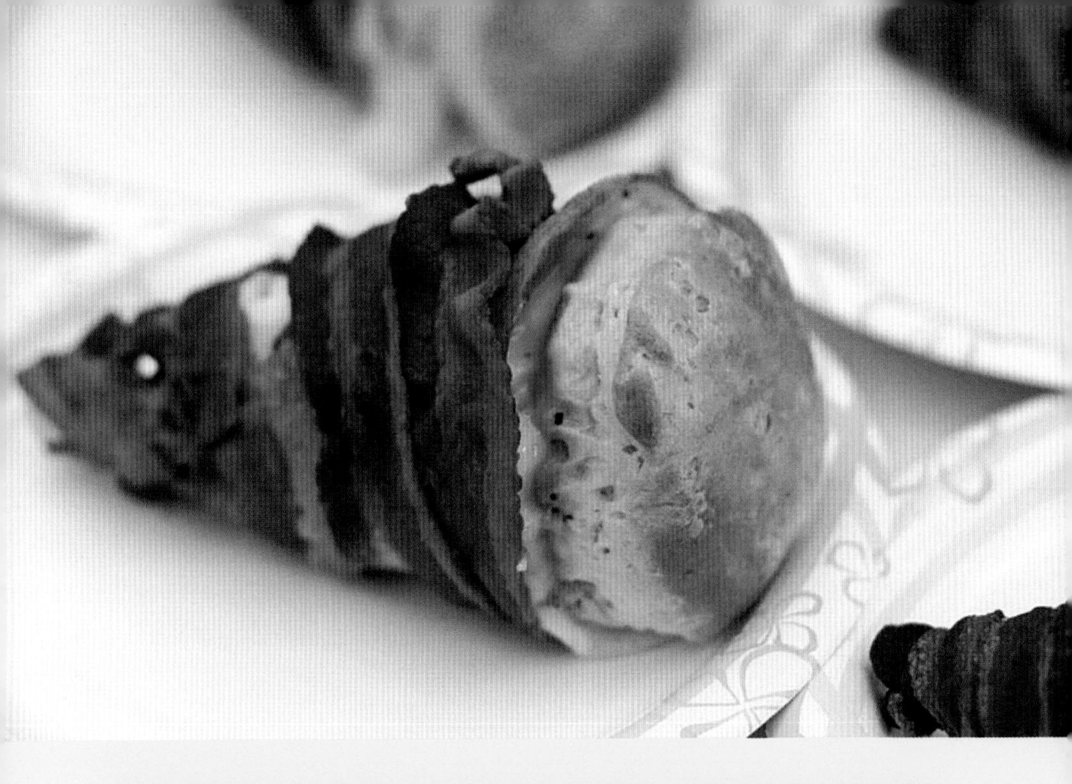

combination of scrambled eggs, hash browns, and cheese. I thought it was a funny idea, but I wasn't sold until Melissa excitedly shouted, "and topped with a biscuit!" That's all it needed. It was the perfect idea and I could see it clearly. This picture of the bacone looks exactly the way I envisioned it that night at the diner. We took it to Bacon Camp, won the judges' choice award, and walked away with an armful of prizes including a bacon wallet and bacon-flavored dental floss!

Bacon Beeritos

Recipe by sheniferous (Flickr)

1 1/2 cups flour
1 tsp paprika
1/8 tsp pepper
12 oz light beer
4 thick-cut bacon strips
1 package bacon bits
2 containers all-malt porter of your choosing
2 flour tortillas
1 package shredded beef
1 can black beans
2 cups cooked rice
4 chopped chilies
2 tbsp cumin
2 tbsp ground cloves
2 tbsp oregano
2 tbsp thyme
1 onion, chopped
1 can corn
1 package shredded pepper Jack, cheddar, and mozzarella cheese mixture

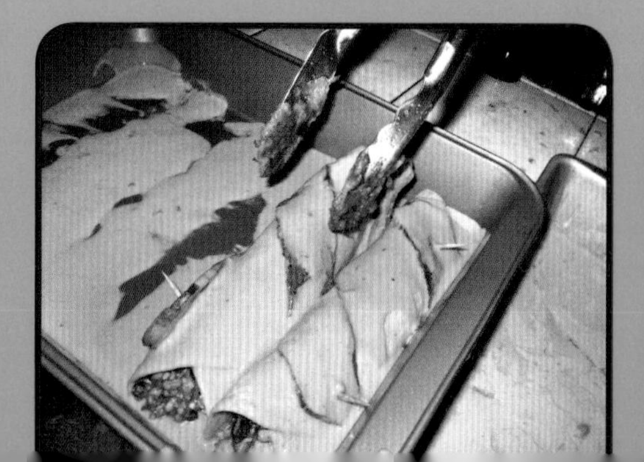

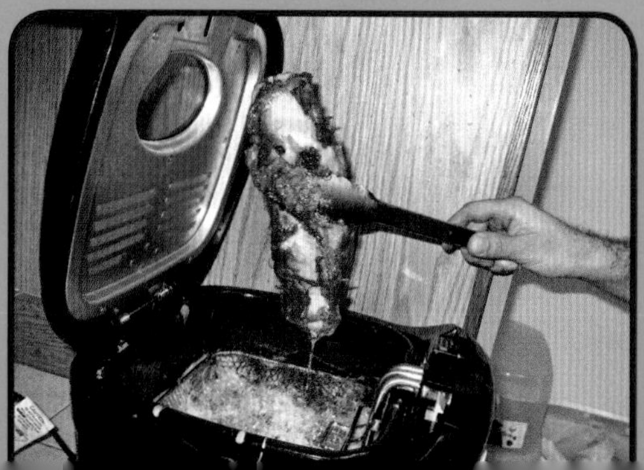

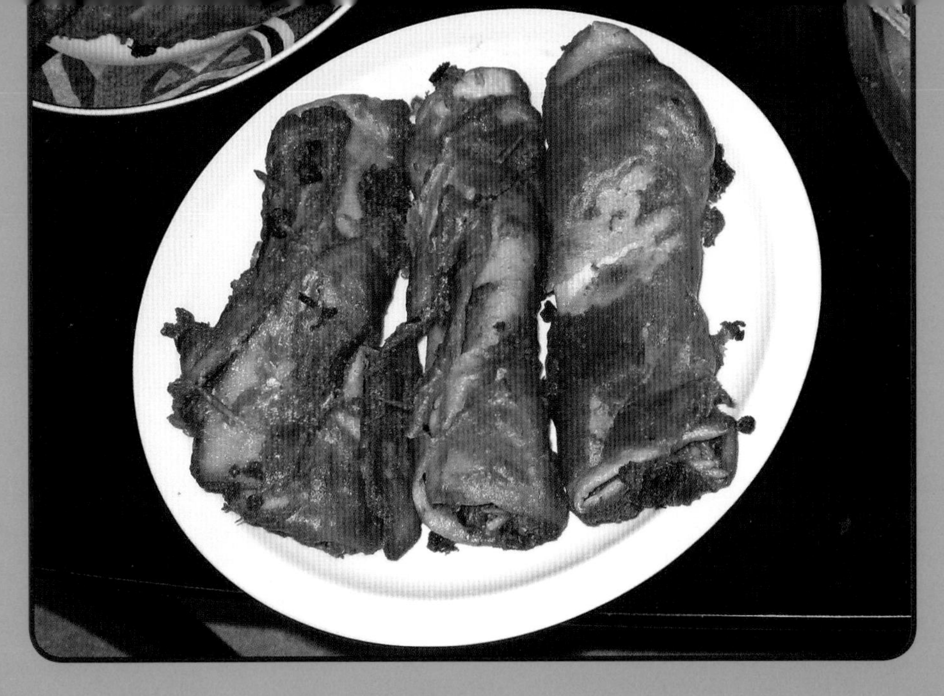

Add the flour, paprika, and pepper to a large bowl. Gradually stir in light beer with a whisk. Beat the batter until it's smooth, and set aside. Bake at 350° F the four thick-cut strips of bacon and a package of bacon bits in an all-malt porter of your choosing. Then soak two tortillas in the porter and let dry. Add porter into the beer batter as well. In a large bowl, mix shredded beef with black beans, rice, chilies, cumin, ground cloves, oregano, thyme, and onion. Then add corn and cheese. Pour the second bottle of all-malt porter directly into the mixture, along with the bacon bits. On a flat surface, put a generous amount of filling onto a tortilla. Wrap it up and then wrap strips of bacon around it. Beer-batter the Bacon Beerito and deep-fry until golden.

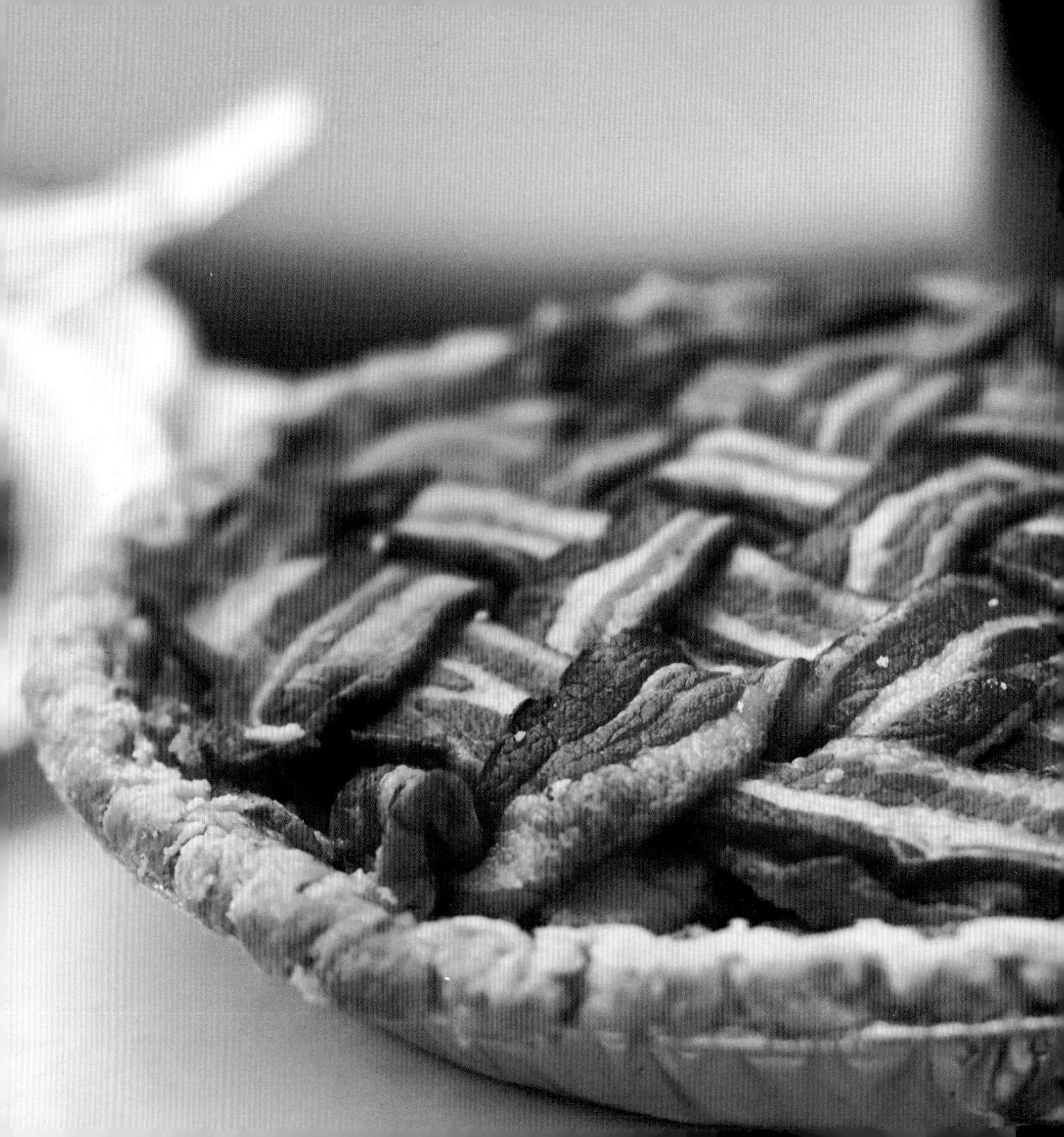

Bacon Apple Pie

Recipe by Phoebe Owens and Michael Crozier

9-inch piecrust
5–6 medium or large tart apples, cored and sliced
1/4 cup dark brown sugar
1 tsp nutmeg
1/2 tbsp cinnamon
2 1/2 tbsp cornstarch
1 tbsp scotch
1/2 cup real maple syrup
6–8 slices bacon

Preheat oven to 350°F. Spread the piecrust on a pan and leave the overhanging edges. Mix the apple slices, brown sugar, nutmeg, cloves, cinnamon, cornstarch, and scotch. Spread over piecrust. Pour the maple syrup evenly over the apples. Arrange the strips of bacon over the top of the piecrust in a lattice, then fold the edges of the piecrust over the bacon and crimp. Bake for 60 minutes, or until the bacon on top is nicely crisp and the crust is browned.

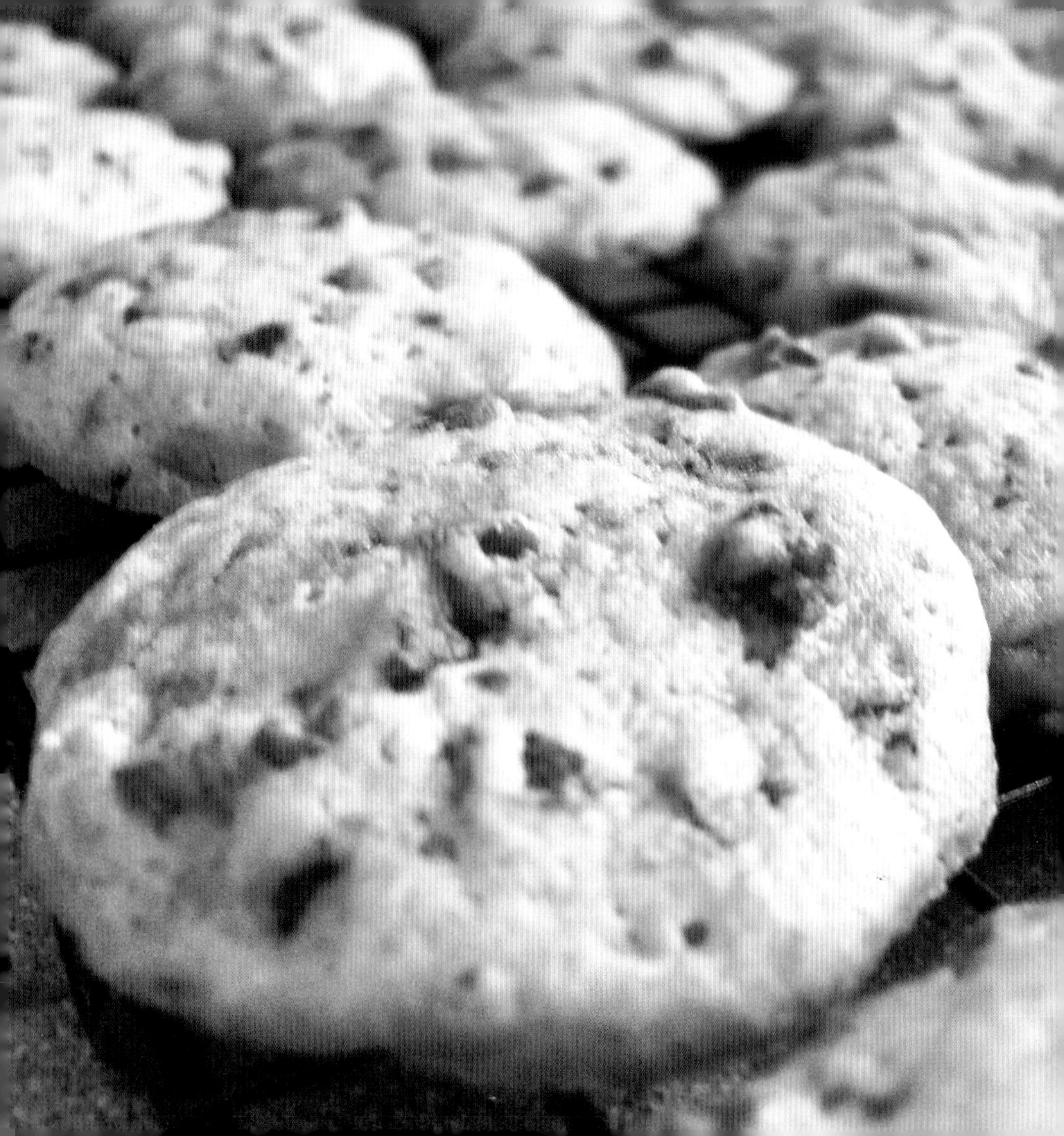

Bacon Chocolate Chip Cookies

Recipe by Maggie Fritz-Morkin

- 5–8 bacon strips
- 1/2 cup butter
- 1/2 cup brown sugar
- 1/4 cup white sugar
- 1/2 tsp vanilla
- 1 egg
- 1/2 tsp sea salt
- 3/4 tsp baking soda
- 1 1/2 cups plus 2 tbsp flour
- 2/3 cup milk chocolate bits

Preheat oven to 375°F. Fry strips of bacon (equivalent to ½ cup chopped) until very crispy. Chop into bits. In a mixer, mix butter, brown sugar, and white sugar into a cream. Mix in the vanilla and the egg. Add the sea salt, baking soda, and flour. Stir in the milk chocolate bits and bits of bacon. Put 1-inch balls of dough on a greased cookie sheet and bake for 10 minutes.

Bacon Explosion Wellington

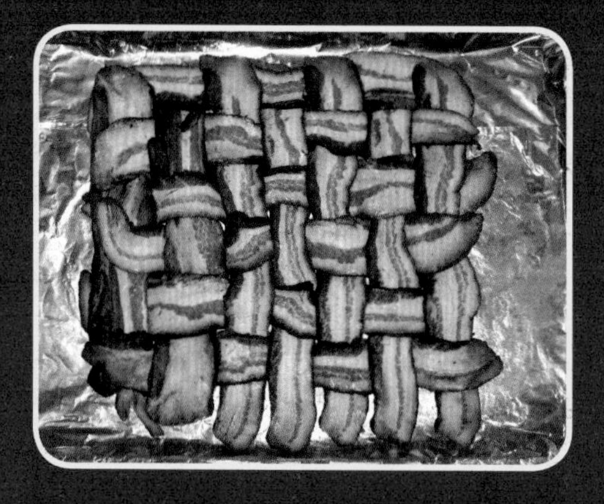

- 2 lbs thick-cut bacon
- 1 jar barbecue seasoning
- 2 lbs Italian sausage
- 1 jar barbecue sauce
- 1 sheet puff pastry, frozen store-bought (11 × 17 inches)
- 1 egg, beaten with a splash of water

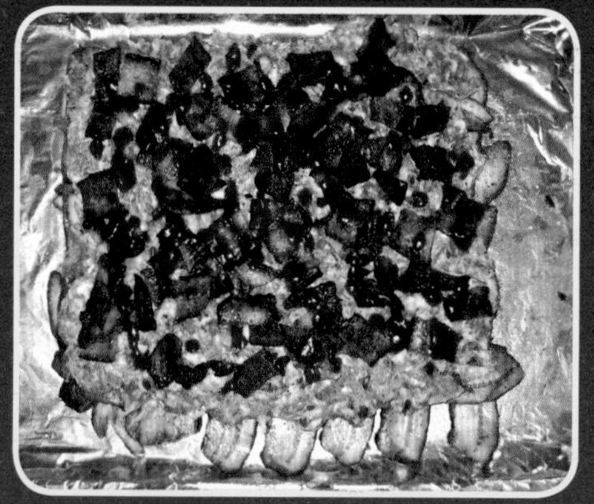

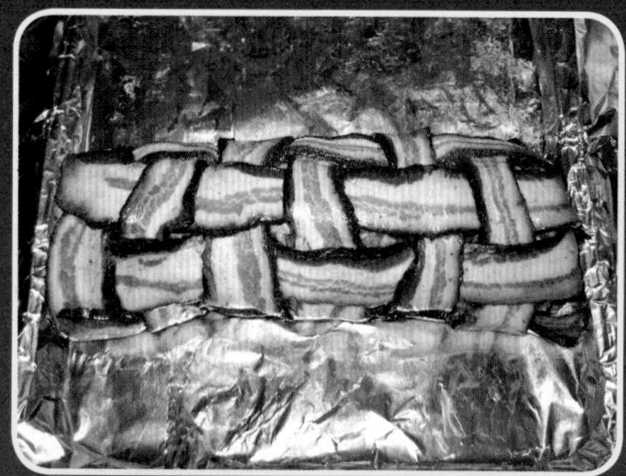

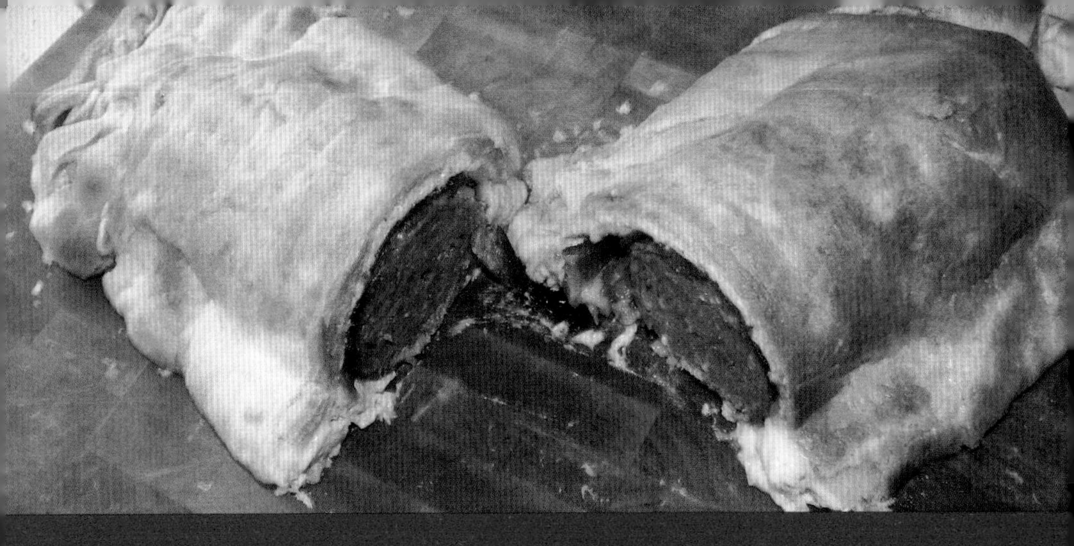

Create a 5 × 5 tight bacon weave. Add barbecue seasoning on top of the bacon weave. Layer the Italian sausage directly on top of the bacon weave. Spread the sausage evenly to the outer edges of the bacon weave. Fry the remaining bacon slices, then chop into bite-size pieces and place on top of the sausage. Add a layer of barbecue sauce and seasoning over the bacon pieces. Very carefully separate the front edge of the sausage layer from the bacon weave and begin rolling backward—rolling all layers but the weave. Once the sausage is fully rolled, pinch together the seams and ends to seal. Roll the sausage forward, completely wrapping it in the bacon weave with the seam facing down. Spread a thick layer of puff pastry onto a cookie sheet covered with parchment paper. Place the bacon explosion in the center and wrap dough up and over the bacon explosion. Trim excess dough and seal with the egg wash, using a pastry brush. Turn the Bacon Explosion Wellington over and cover with the egg wash. Place a thermometer into the thickest part of the meat. Bake in a roasting pan at 375°F for 1 hour, or until the internal temperature reads 165°F and the outer layer is golden brown.

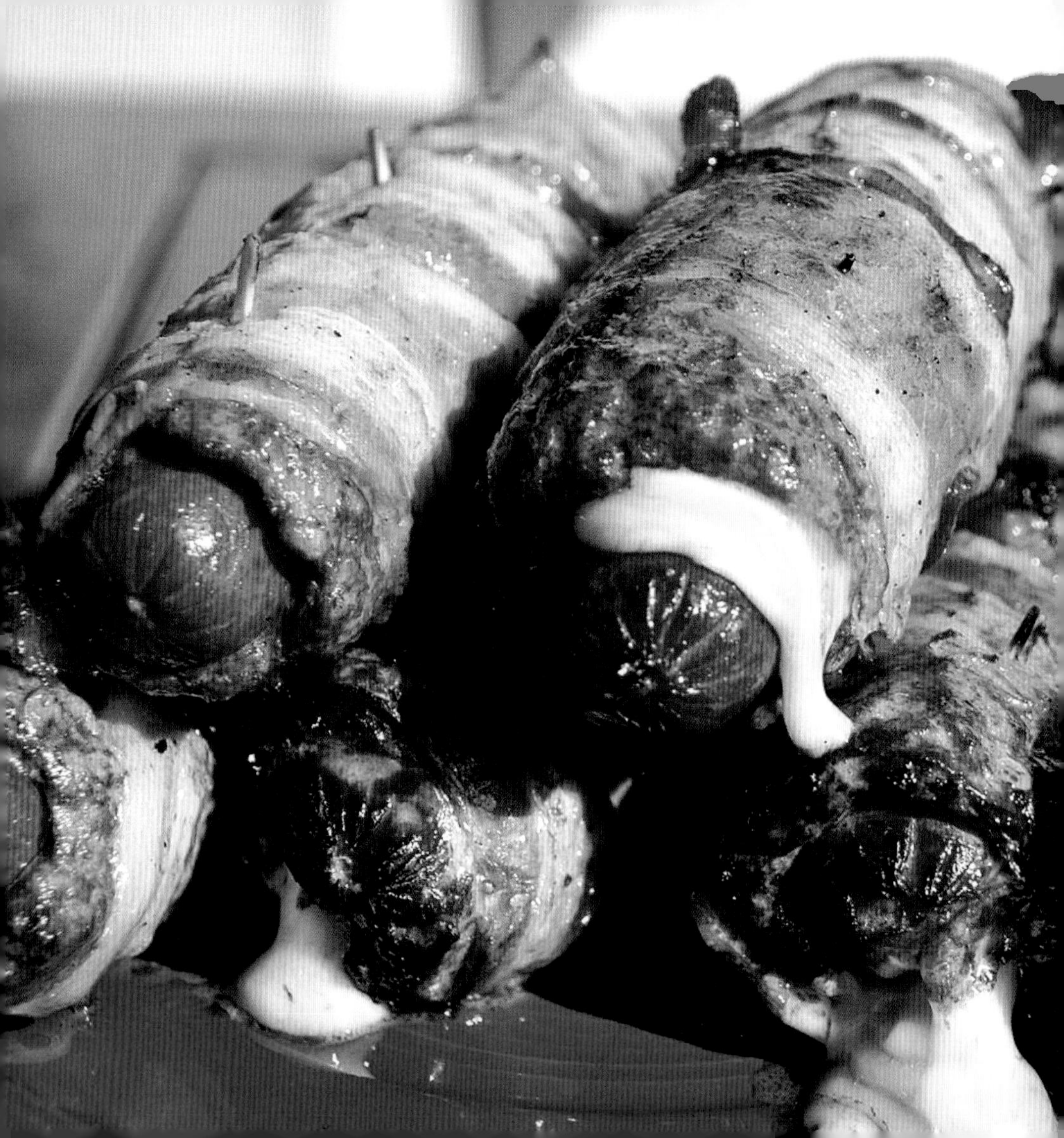

Bacon Burger Dog

Recipe by Texas Burger Guy

6–8 oz ground beef
1 hot dog
2 bacon strips
4–5 slices of American cheese
1 roll
Ketchup and/or mustard

Spread ground beef flat in the shape of a square, slightly shorter than a hot dog. Layer slices of cheese across ground beef. Place a hot dog on the beef and roll it up. Press the beef together so the hot dog is completely wrapped up, leaving the ends of the dog sticking out. Wrap the burger-dog combo in two strips of bacon. Grill for 20 to 30 minutes over medium heat. Place the burger dog on a roll and top with ketchup and/or mustard to taste.

Bacon Weave Cheese Roll-up

Recipe by erdero (Flickr)

20 bacon strips

1 bag shredded cheddar cheese

Weave bacon together (10 × 10 strips) as tightly as possible. Next, sprinkle with shredded cheese and roll up the bacon weave. Bake at 350°F. Slice and serve.

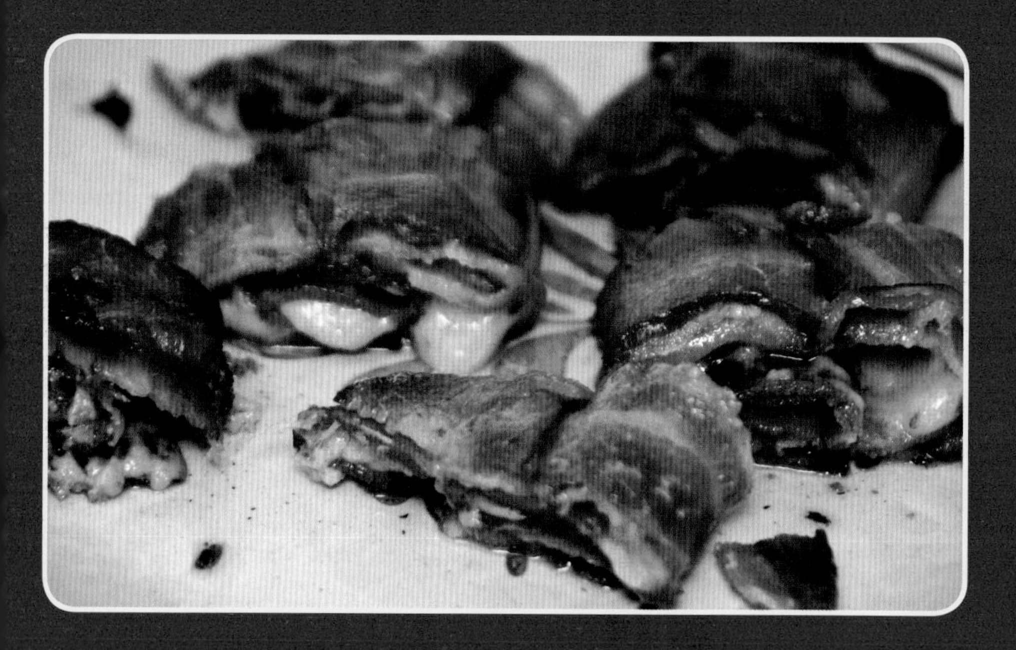

Chocolate-Covered Bacon

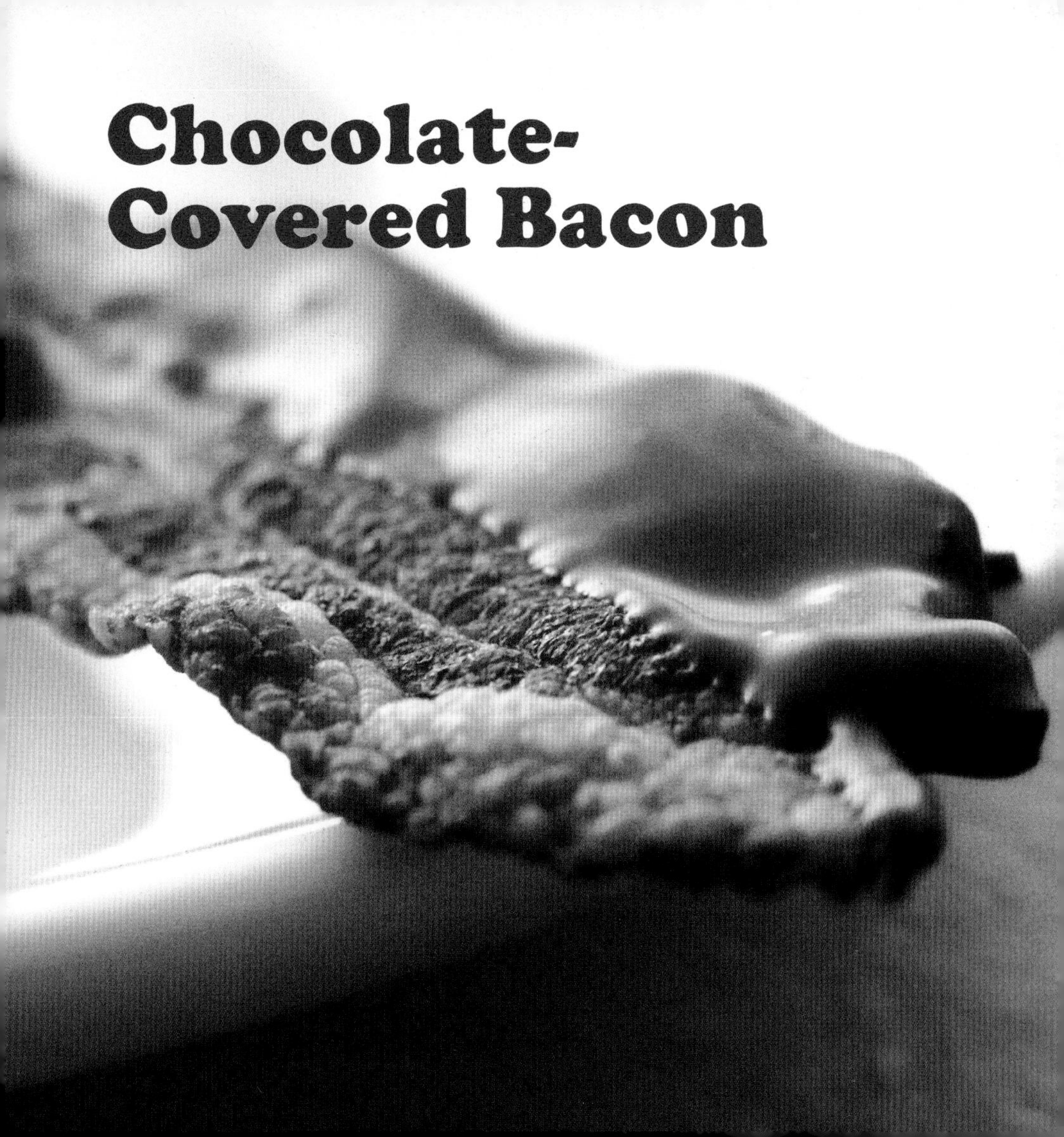

LOCAL FAVE!

Yo Mama's
New Orleans, LA

Peanut Butter Bacon Burger

Souped-up Sandwiches

29,559 Calorie Sandwich

Recipe by Josh Mattson

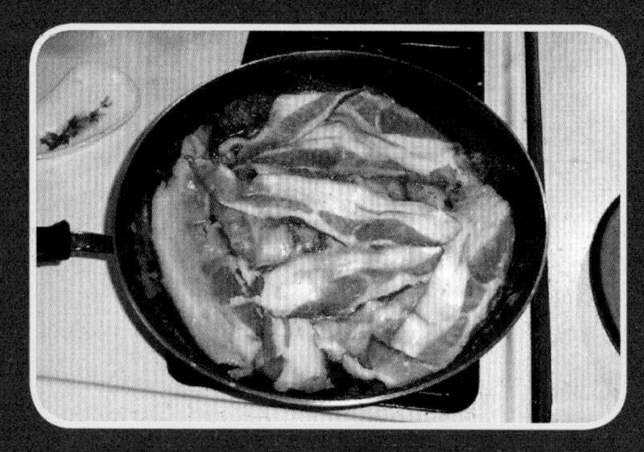

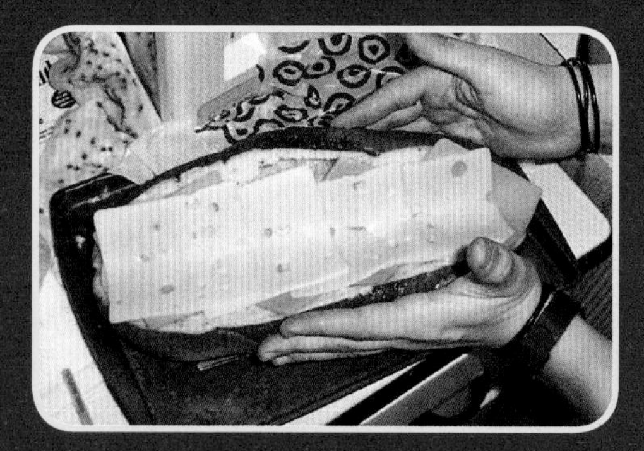

- 15 fried mushrooms (450)
- 14 bacon slices (990)
- 18 onion rings (1140)
- 1/4 lb ground beef (293)
- 2 corn dogs (540)
- 4 slices Swiss cheese (425)
- 4 slices provolone cheese (397)
- 4 slices cheddar cheese (455)
- 1/4 lb sliced ham (184)
- 1/4 lb sliced turkey (181)
- 1/4 lb pastrami (394)
- 1/4 lb sliced roast beef (200)
- 1 bratwurst (510)
- 1/4 lb braunschweiger (580)
- 1 lb wheat bread (1030)

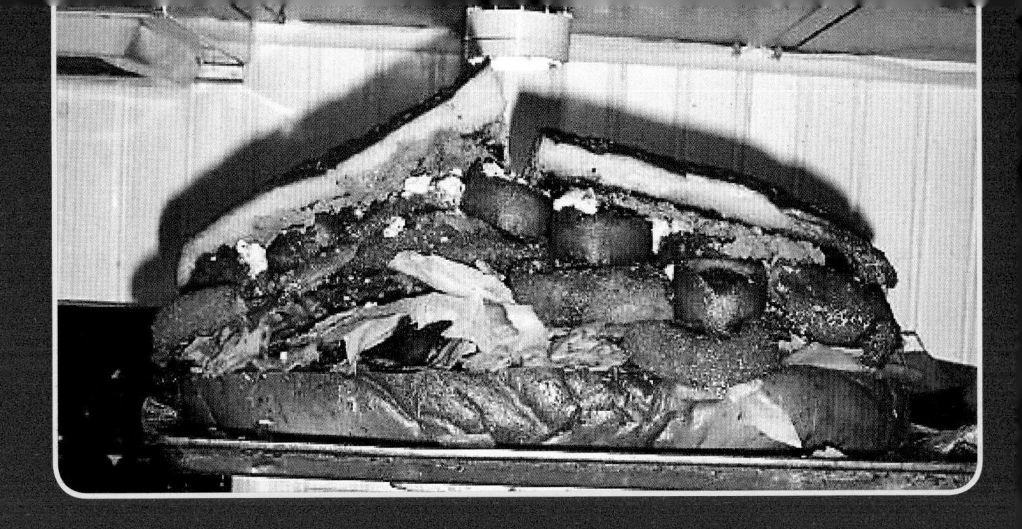

½ head lettuce (25)
4 oz feta cheese (350)
6 oz Italian salad dressing (480)
1.75 oz oregano (438)
1.75 oz salt (0)
½ lb butter (1600)
3.5 oz Parmesan cheese (465)
9.5 cups canola oil (18,432)

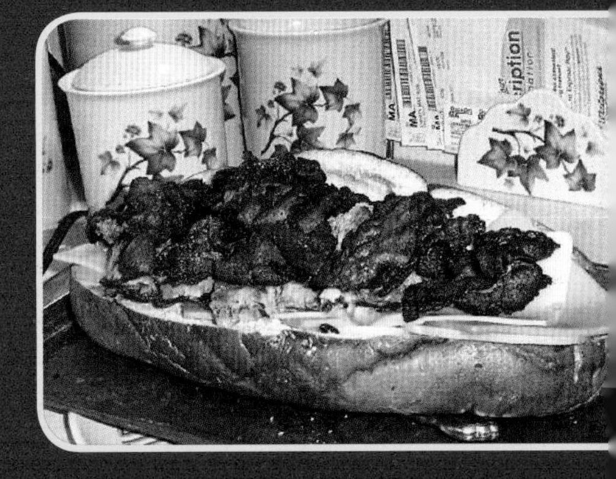

Total: 29,559 calories

Kenny & Zuke's DDD Reuben

LOCAL FAVE!
Kenny & Zuke's
Portland, OR

A deep-fried triple-decker Reuben, featuring four slices of rye, loads of kraut and Russian dressing, a quarter pound of Swiss, all over a pound of pastrami.

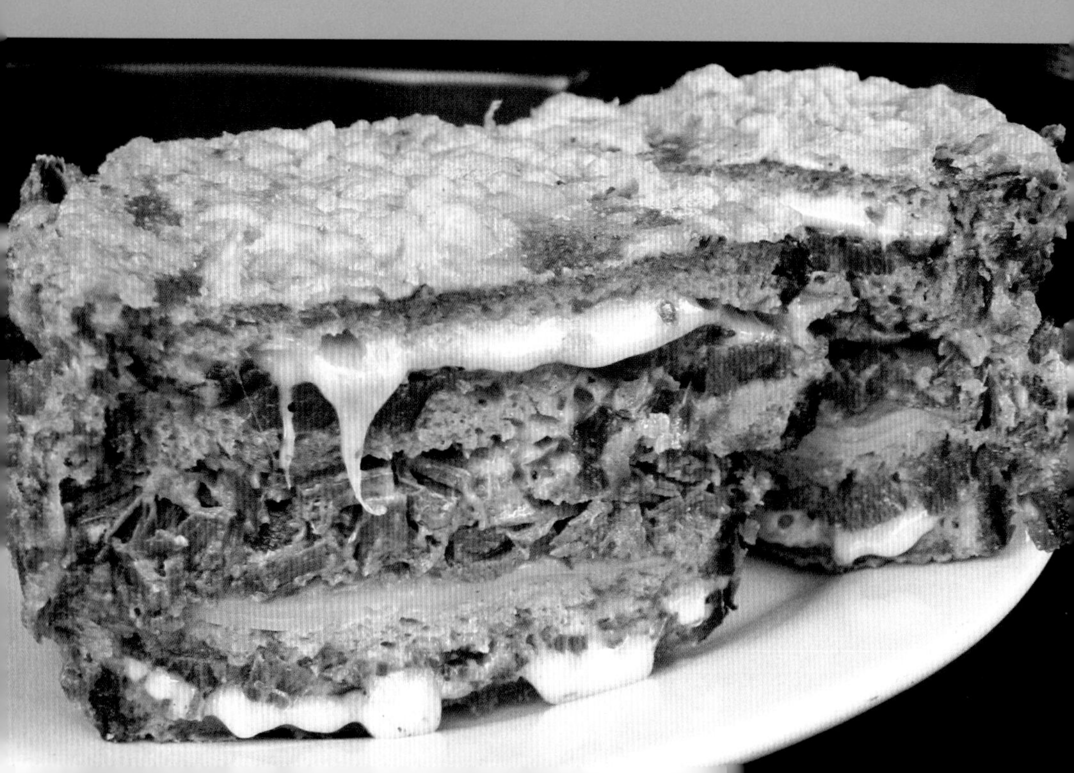

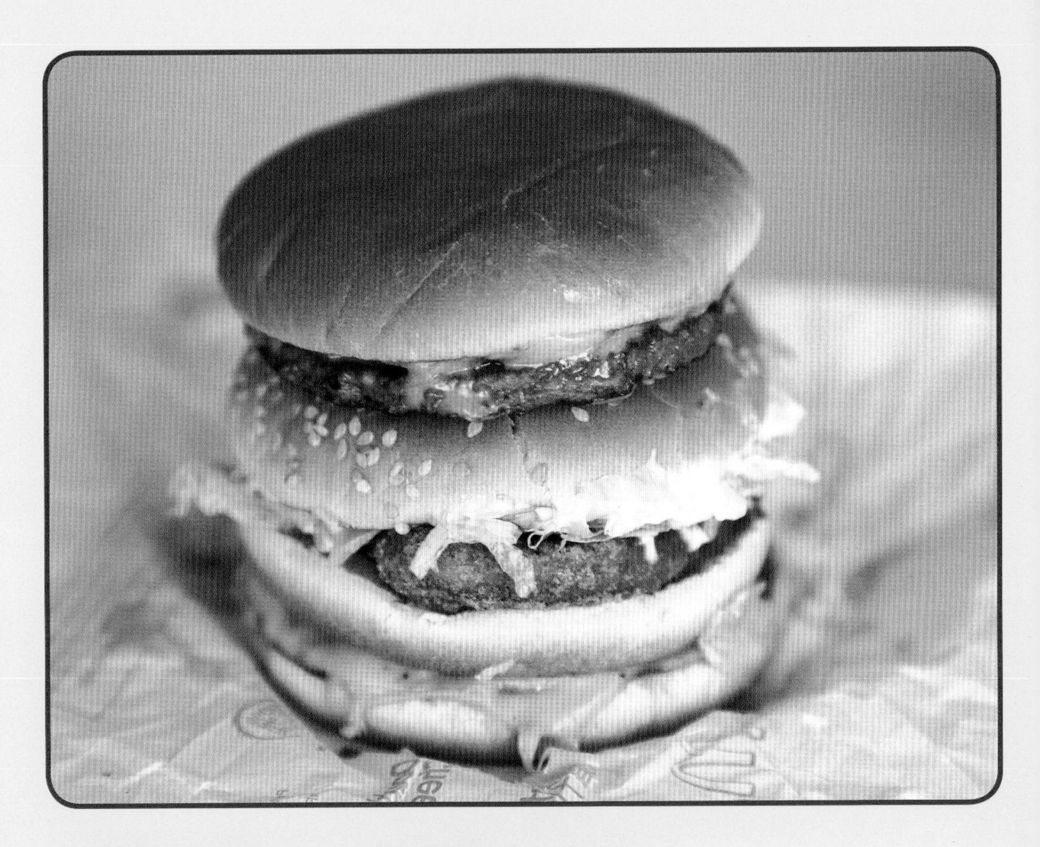

McGangBang

A McChicken sandwich inside a double cheeseburger.

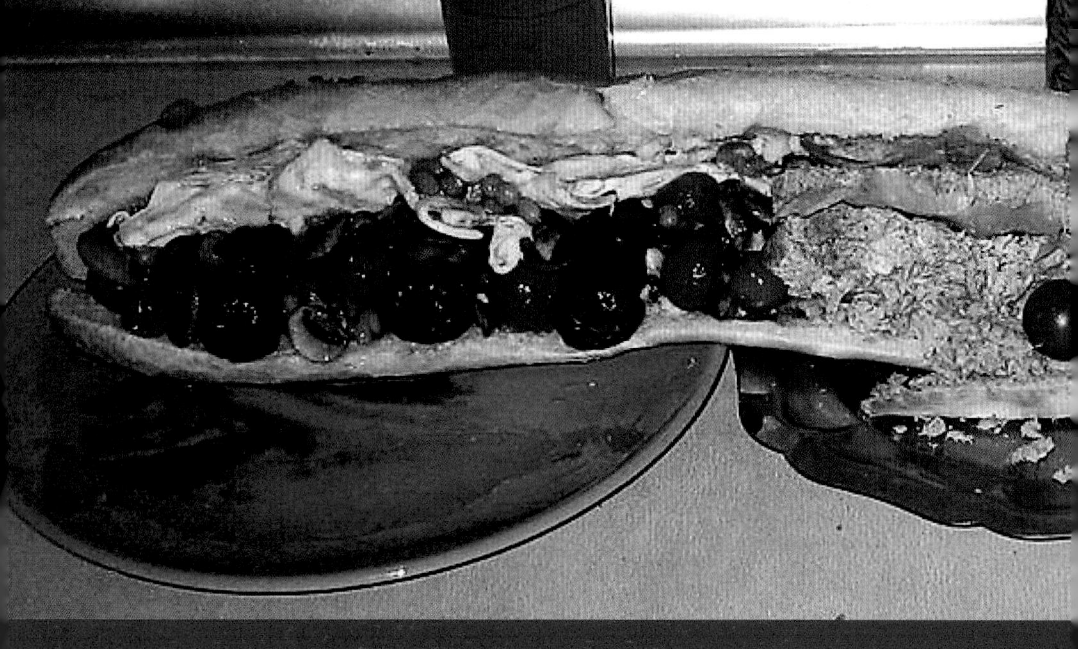

All-Day-Long Sandwich of Dreams

Recipe by Rosa, Paul, and Tara

Breakfast Section:
Sausages, baked beans, bacon, grilled tomatoes, mushrooms, and multiple fried eggs

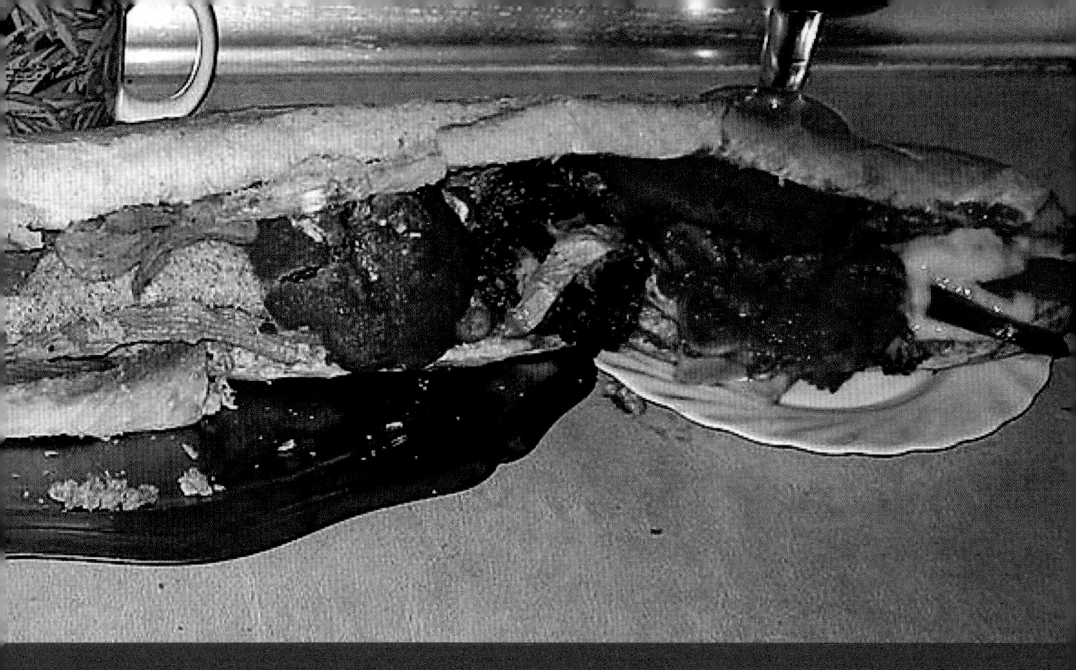

Lunch Section:

Tuna and mayonnaise sandwich, cherry tomato garnish, and potato chips

Afternoon Tea Section:

Scone, jam (strawberry), and cream

Aperitif Section:

Olives (stuffed with anchovies)

Dinner Section:

Lasagna, fish sticks, and broccoli

Dessert Section:

Crème Catalan

Gluttonator

From top to bottom: a bread slice, fried eggs with Worcestershire sauce, a bread slice, breaded chicken breast, a bread slice, onion rings and mayonnaise, a bread slice, sausages with brown sauce, a bread slice, garlic-fried mushrooms with chips and melted cheddar, a bread slice, bacon and tomato sauce, and another slice of bread.

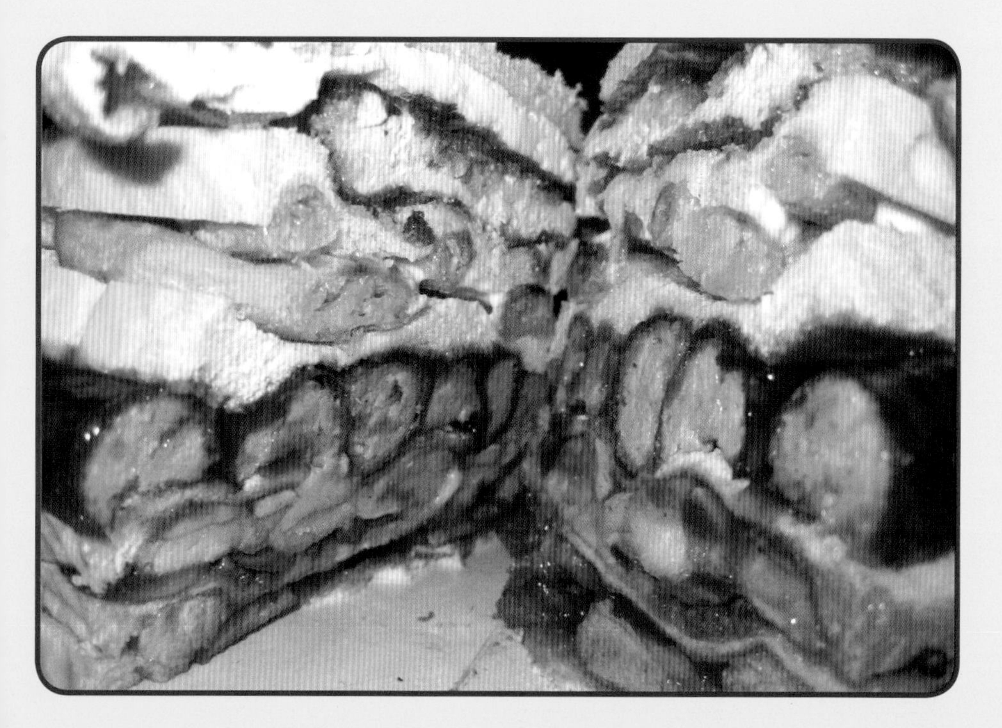

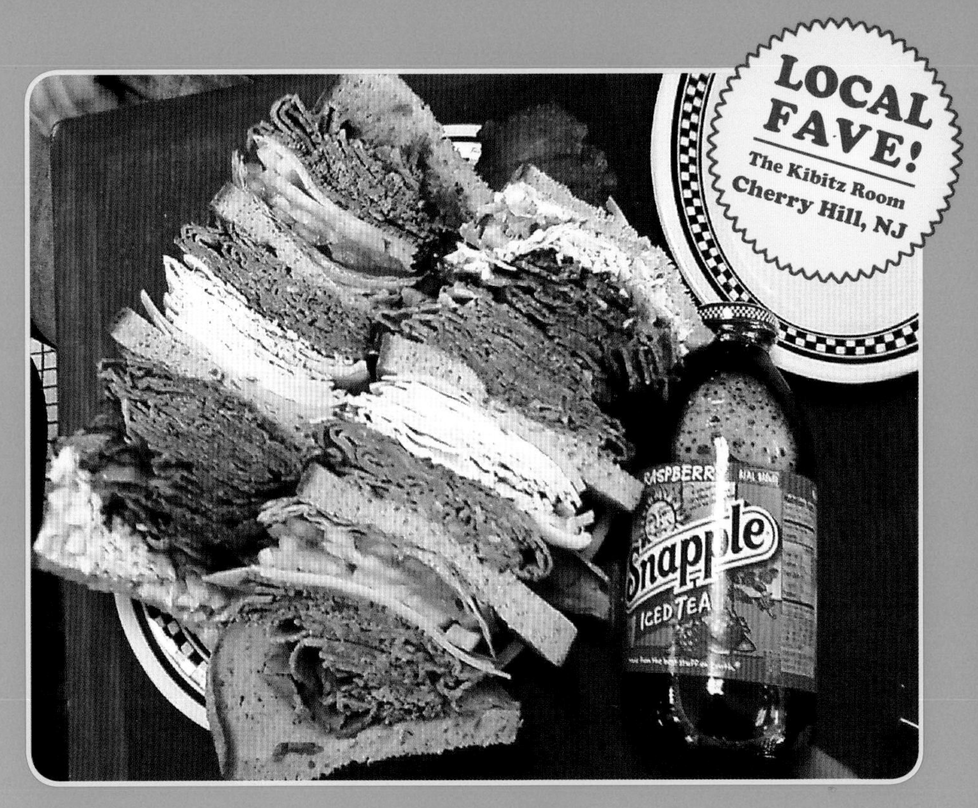

The G.B.M.F.

Corned beef, pastrami, turkey, roast beef, and brisket with cole slaw, Russian dressing, Swiss cheese, lettuce, tomato, and onion.

The American Dream

Recipe by Nick Amosson

Layers from bottom to top:

Pancake
Eggs
Bacon
Sausage
Hash browns
Cheese
Pancake
Pizza
Onion rings
Jalapeño poppers
Cheeseburger
Mozzarella sticks
Pizza
Garlic bread
Mashed potatoes
1 steak
Pasta and meatballs
Garlic bread
4 lbs shredded cheese

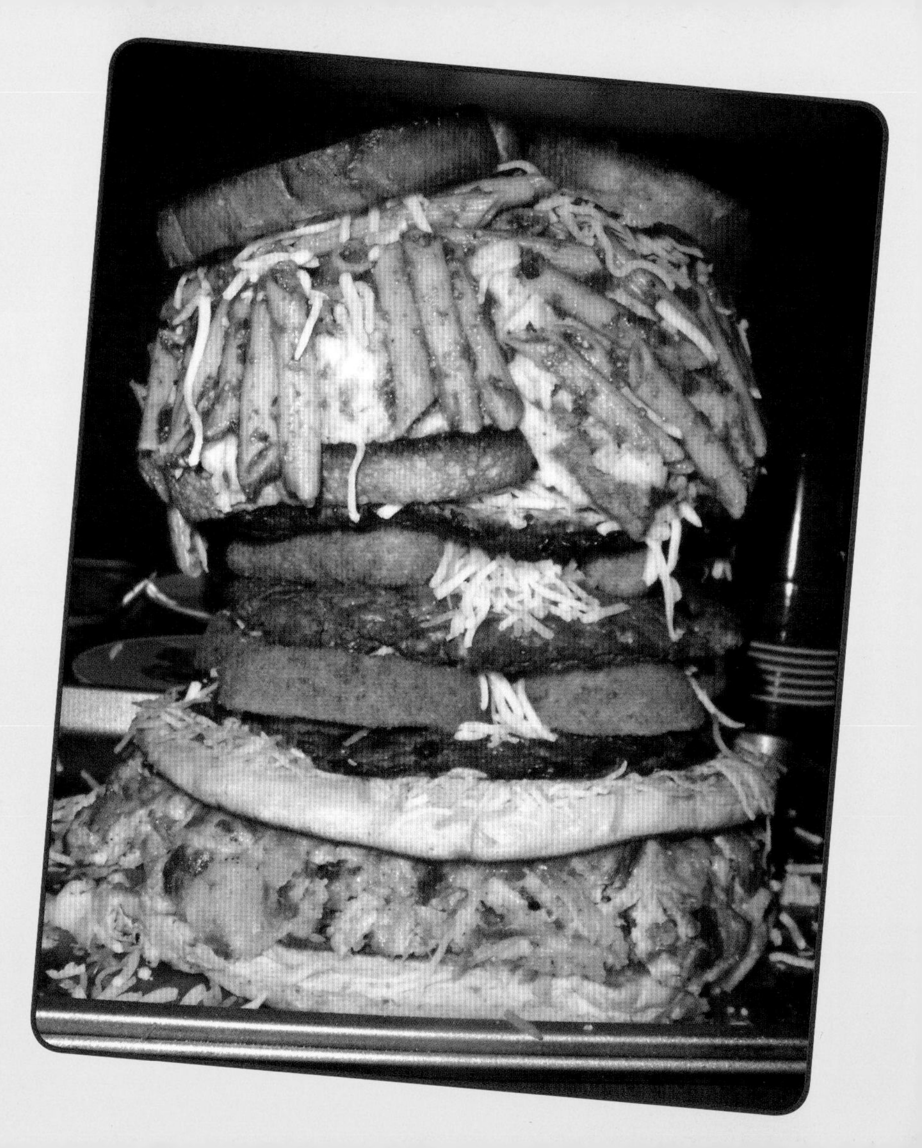

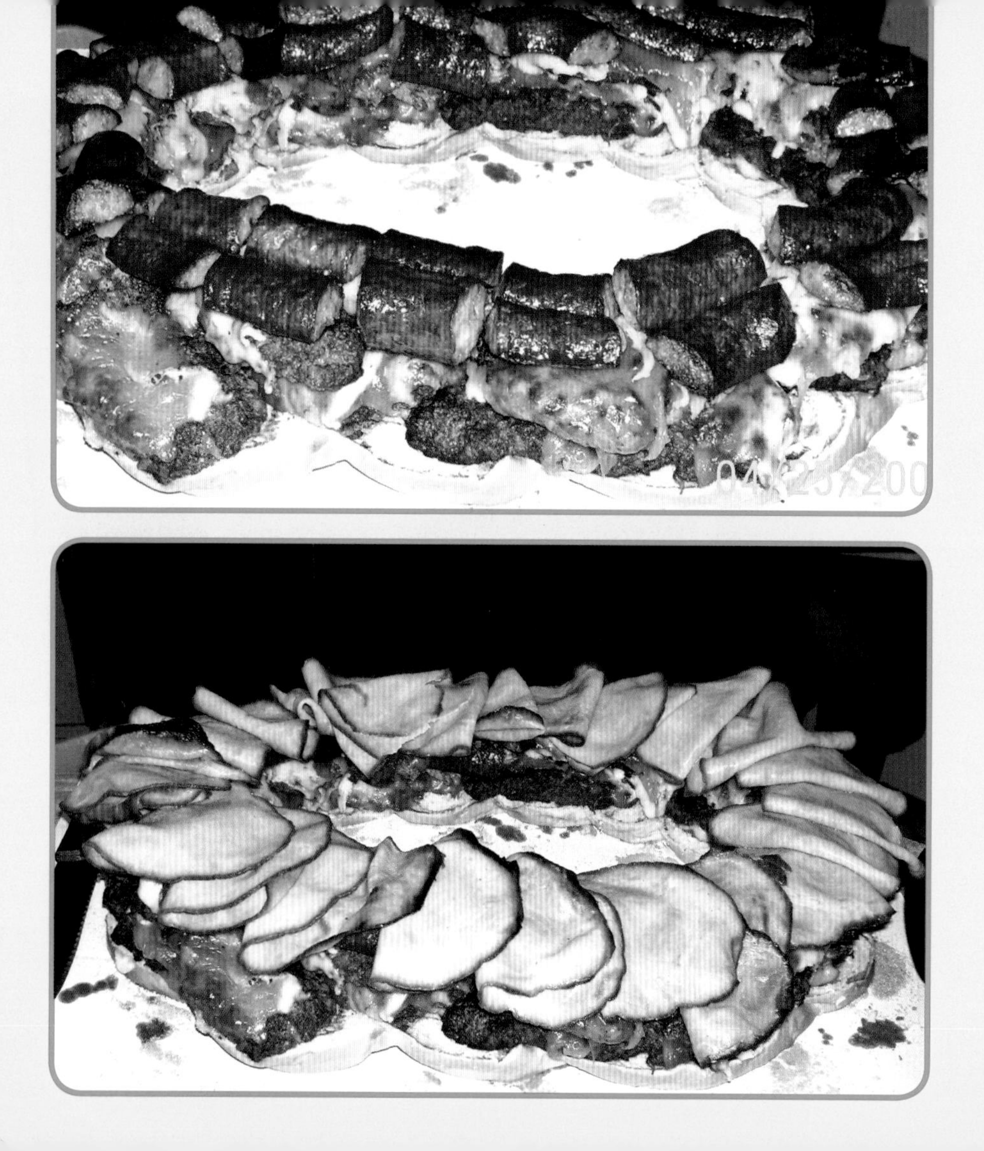
04/25/200

The Fat Tuesday

Recipe by Bryan S. Thompson

Layer One:
Bottom slice of a whole King Cake

Layer Two:
25 cooked cheeseburger patties

Layer Three:
10 sausages, cut in half horizontally, and then sliced vertically

Layer Four:
25 slices of ham, each folded in half, layered over the sausages

Layer Five:
Top slice of the whole King Cake

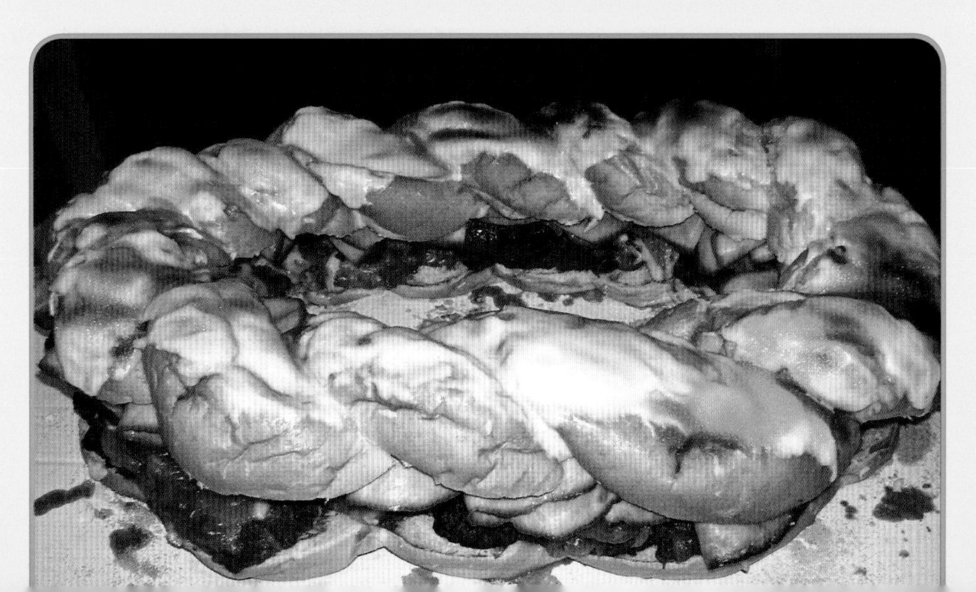

Deep-Fried Grilled-Cheese Sandwich

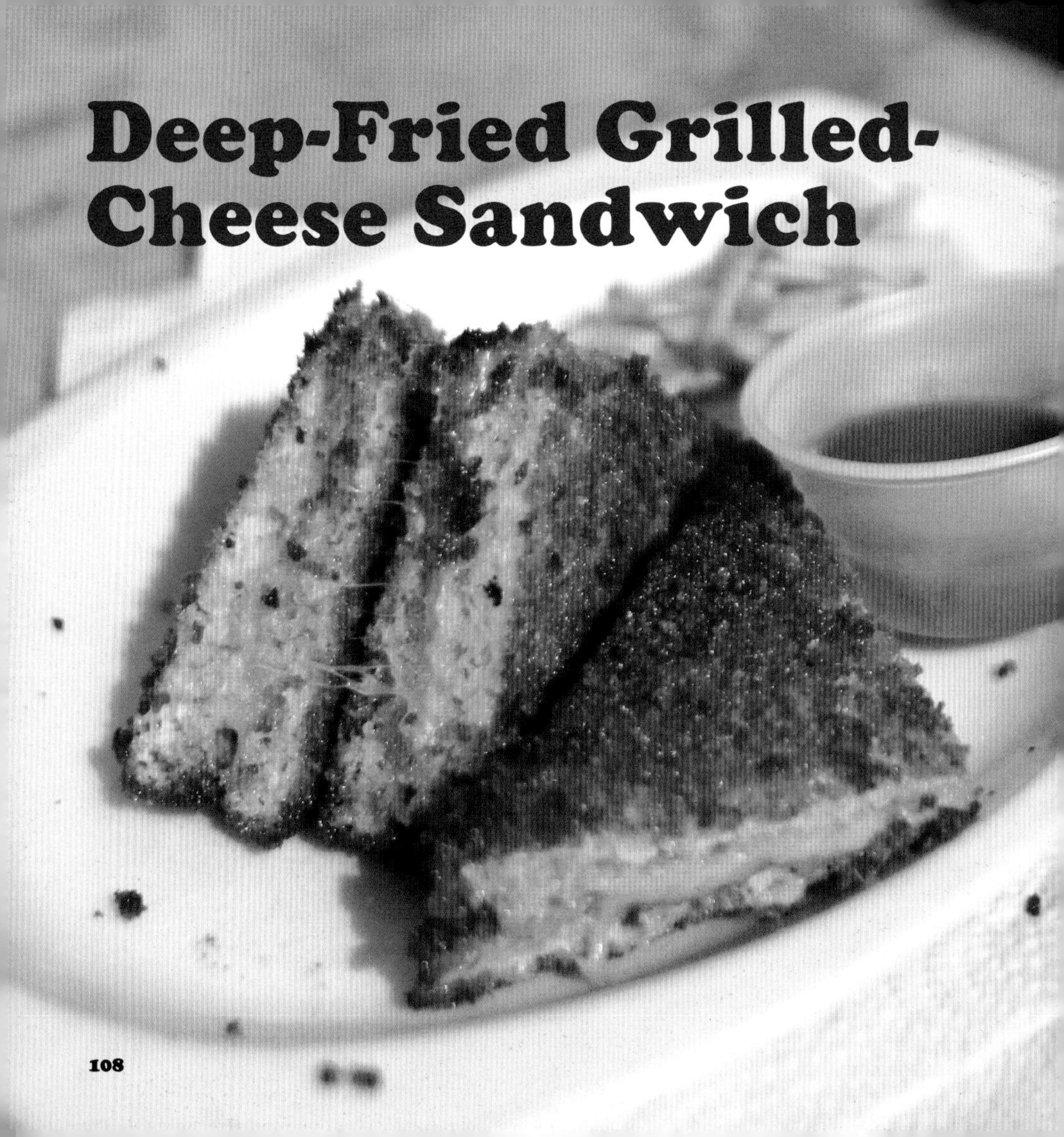

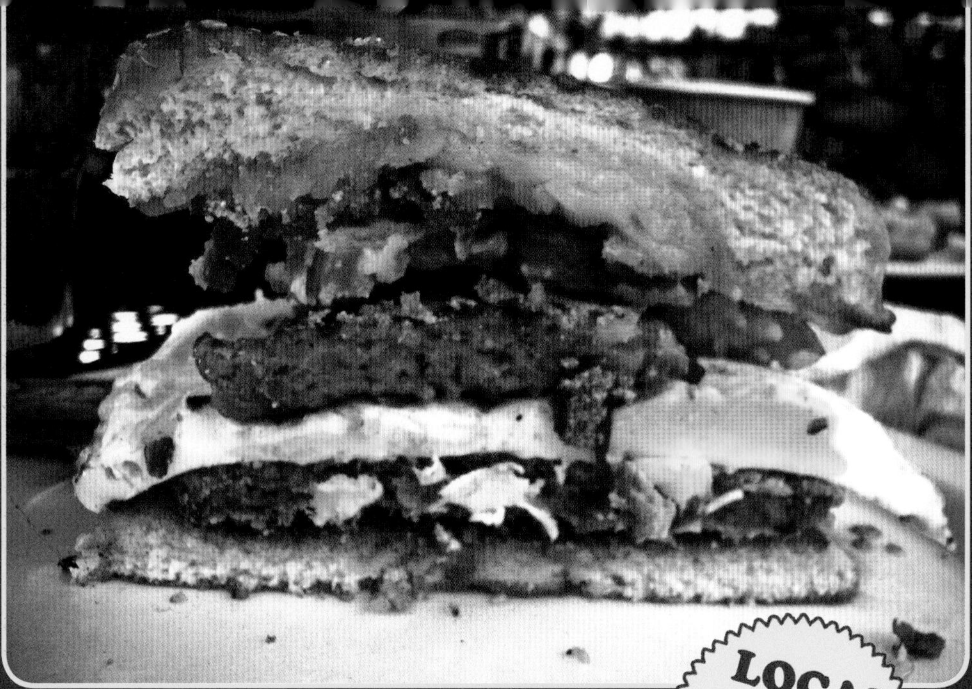

LOCAL FAVE!
Smoky Mountain BBQ
Portland, OR

Heart Attack Sandwich

Chicken-fried steak, chicken-fried bacon, a country sausage, a fried egg, a fried green tomato topped with cheddar cheese and sandwiched between buns fried in bacon fat, all served with a gravy dipping sauce.

Sandwich of Knowledge

Recipe by Luke Berryman

BOTTOM TIER:

Bottom horizontal slice of white bread loaf

8 bacon strips

8 pork sausages

4 $^{1}/_{4}$-lb beef burger patties

1 horizontal slice of white bread loaf

MIDDLE TIER:

1 black pudding sausage, sliced

1 horizontal slice of white bread loaf

TOP TIER:

6 eggs

2 chicken breasts, diced

Top horizontal slice of white bread loaf

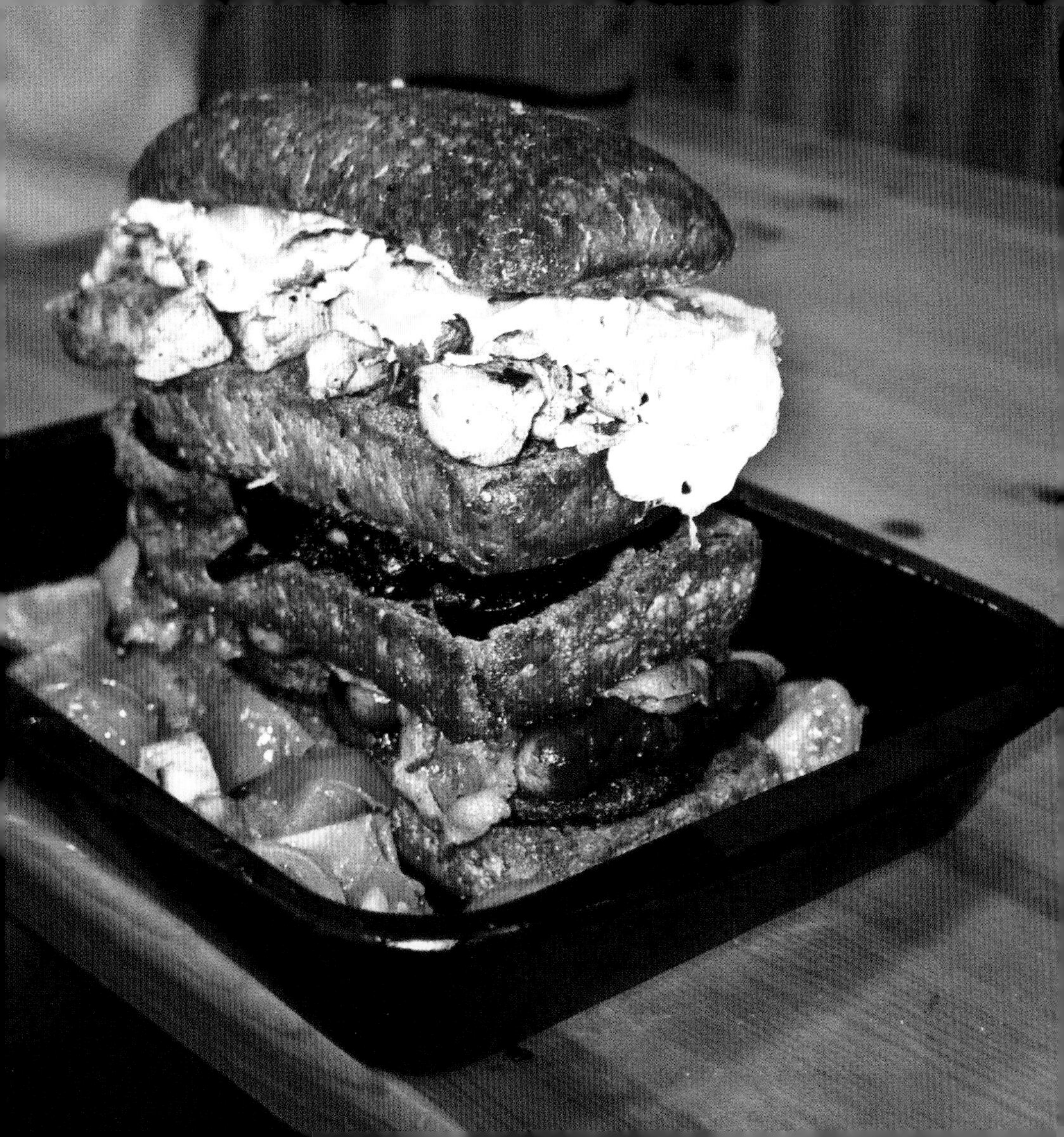

Monster Sandwich Pie

Recipe by Stephen Dietz

1 King's Hawaiian original round loaf
1 container cream cheese
1/2 lb Swiss cheese
1/2 lb cheddar cheese
16 oz onion and chive sour cream
3/4 lb ham
3/4 lb roast beef
3/4 lb turkey
Lettuce
1 tomato
1 onion, thinly sliced
Oil and vinegar
Pepper

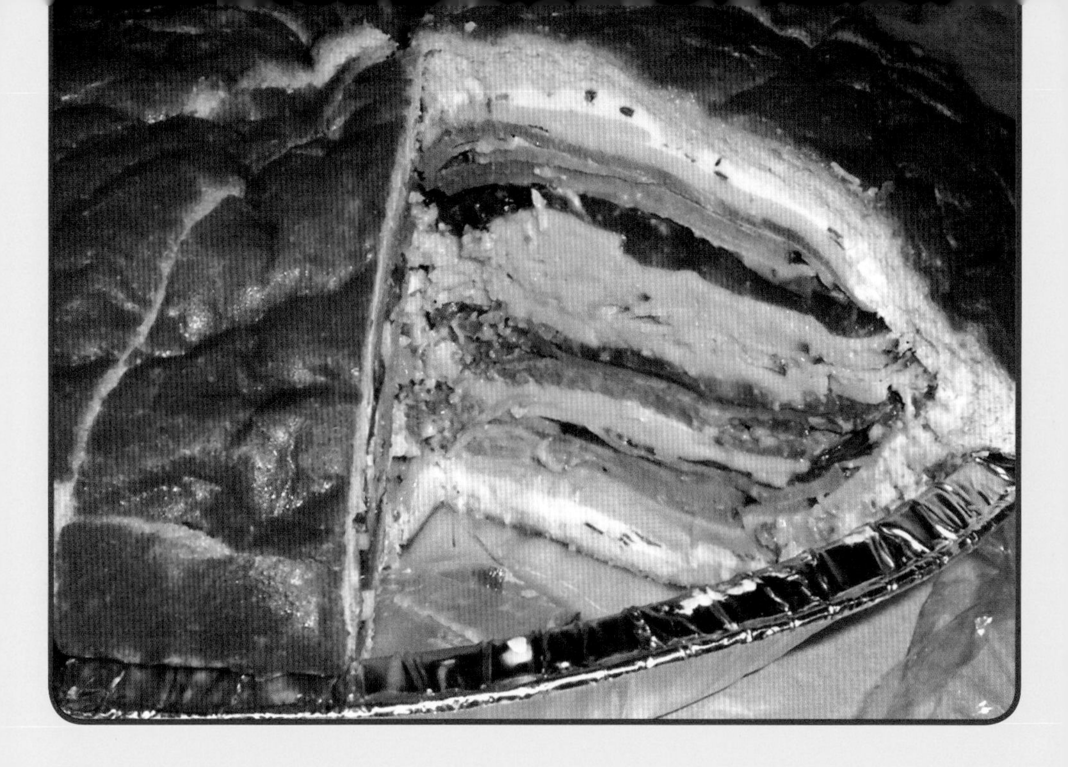

Cut off the top of the loaf right at the rim and set aside. Gut all bread out of the loaf, leaving a shell. Cover the inside and the top with a thick layer of cream cheese. Add remaining cheeses and sour cream, letting the first layer come up on all sides. Next, add layers of one of the meats, lettuce, tomato, and onion, and top with a light dripping of oil and vinegar, then sprinkle on pepper. Repeat this process using different meats with each layer until packed to the top. When the layers have reached the top of the pie, place the top of the loaf back in its original place. Cut as you would a pie.

Big-time Burgers

Luther Burger

A bacon-cheddar cheeseburger with Krispy Kreme donuts as buns.

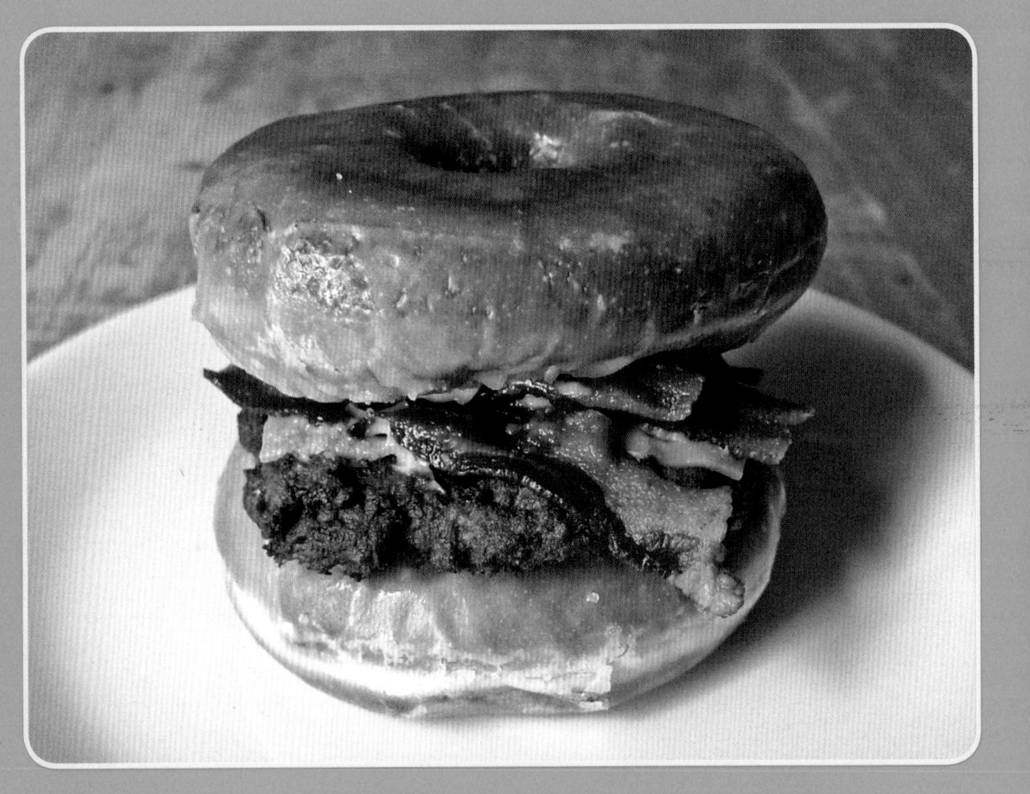

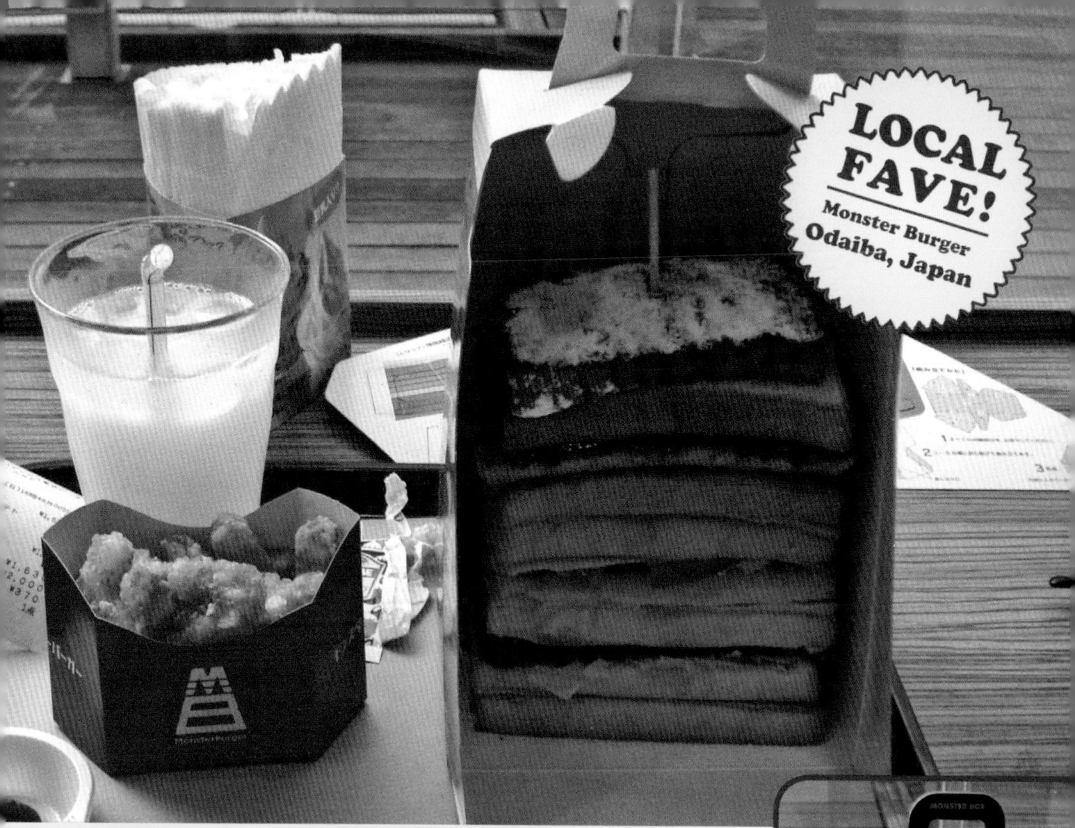

LOCAL FAVE!

Monster Burger
Odaiba, Japan

Monster Box

A skewered sandwich/burger made up of a powdered French toast dessert, a chicken sandwich, a salad sandwich, and a hamburger.

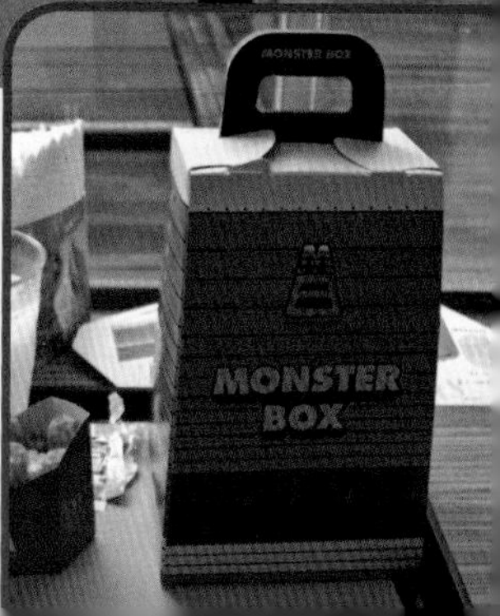

MONSTER BOX

Shake Shack Double Stack

A deep-fried cheese-stuffed portobello mushroom between two cheeseburgers.

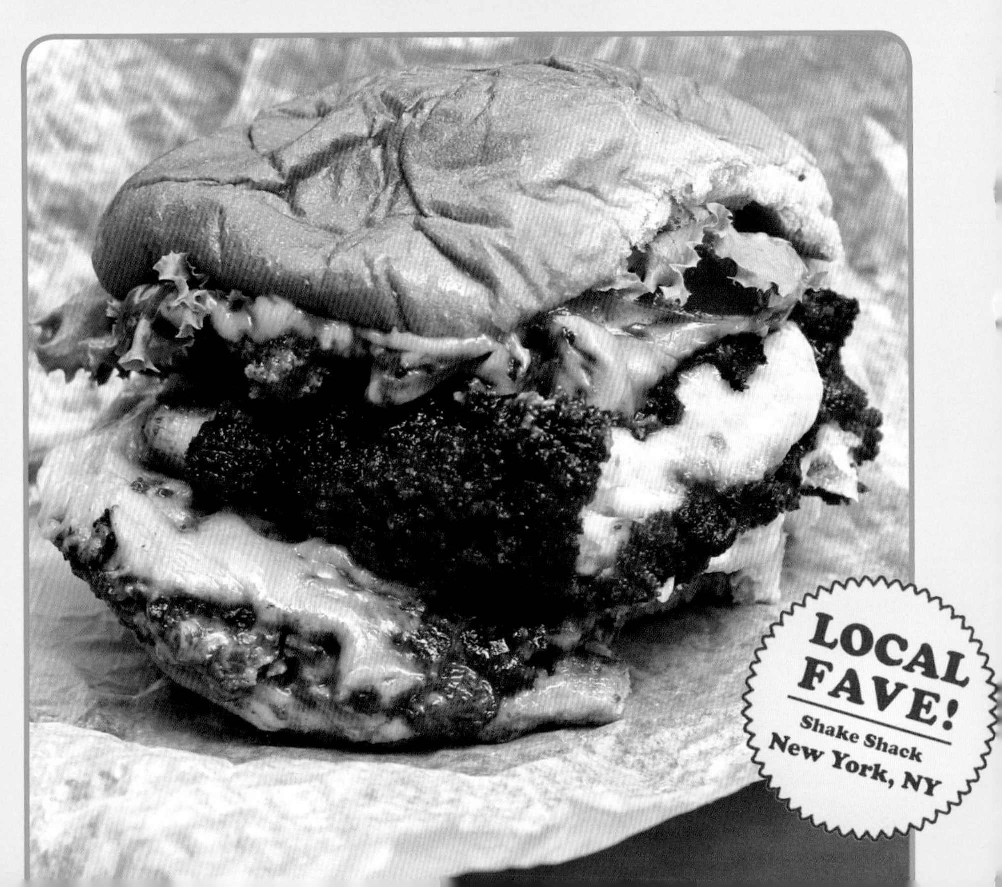

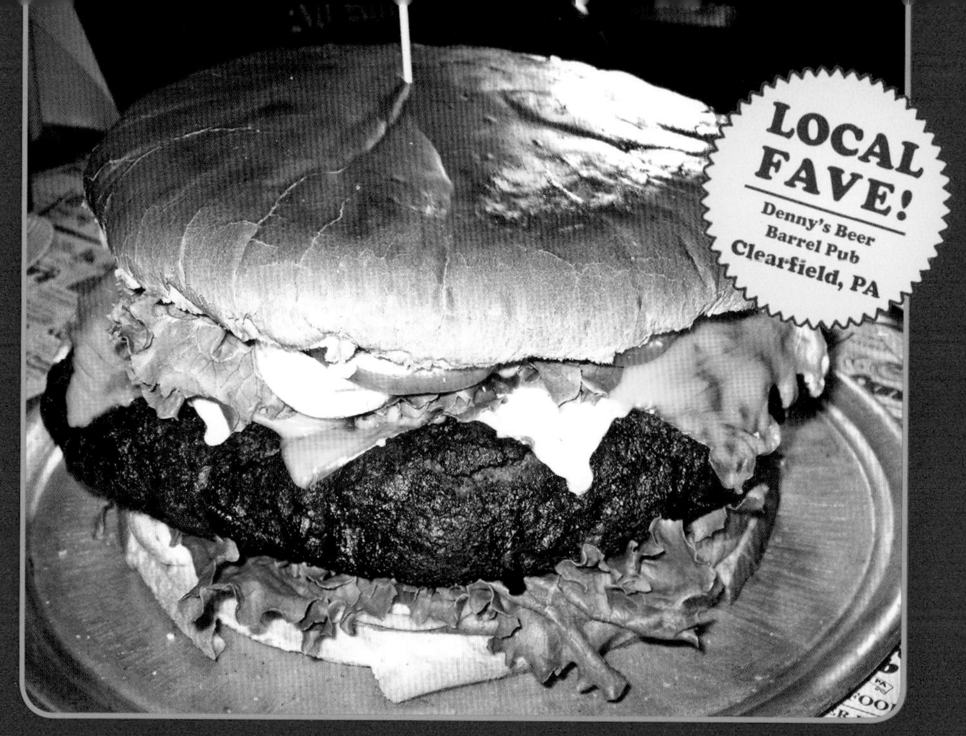

The Beer Barrel Belly Buster

A baked bun, 11 pounds of beef, 25 slices American cheese, 1 head of lettuce, 3 tomatoes, 2 onions, mayo, relish, ketchup, mustard, and banana peppers, garnished with a dozen pickle spears.

Lucy Juicy

A cheeseburger with the cheese cooked inside the burger patty.

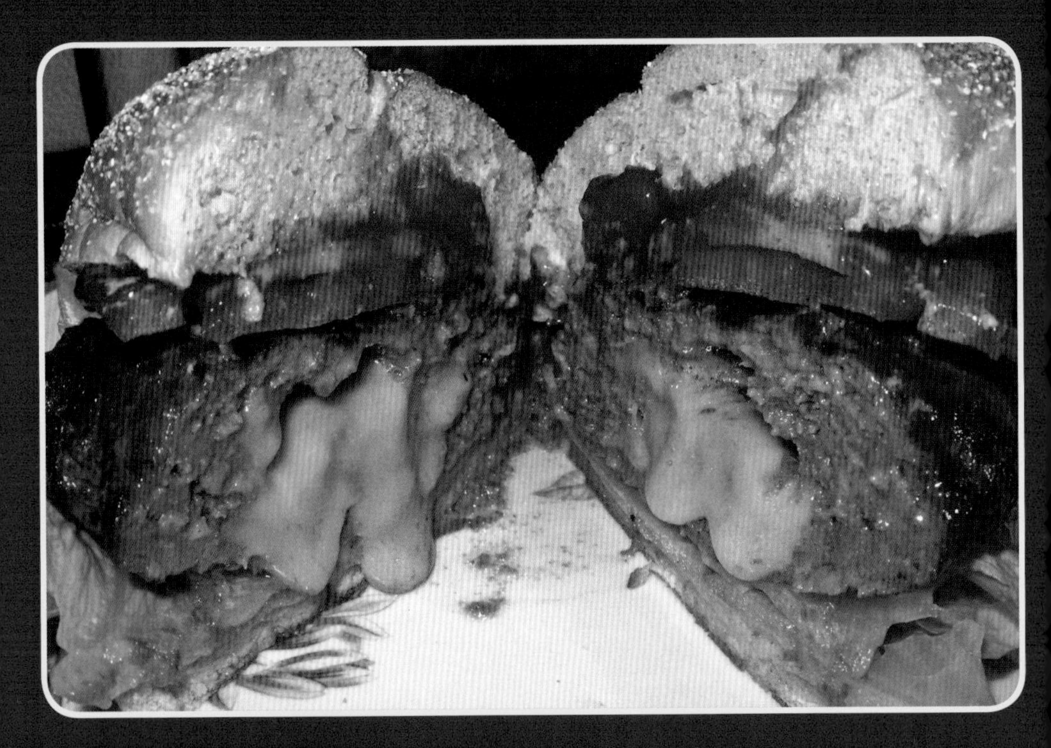

The Squeeze with Cheese

One-third pound of beef smothered in fried cheddar cheese.

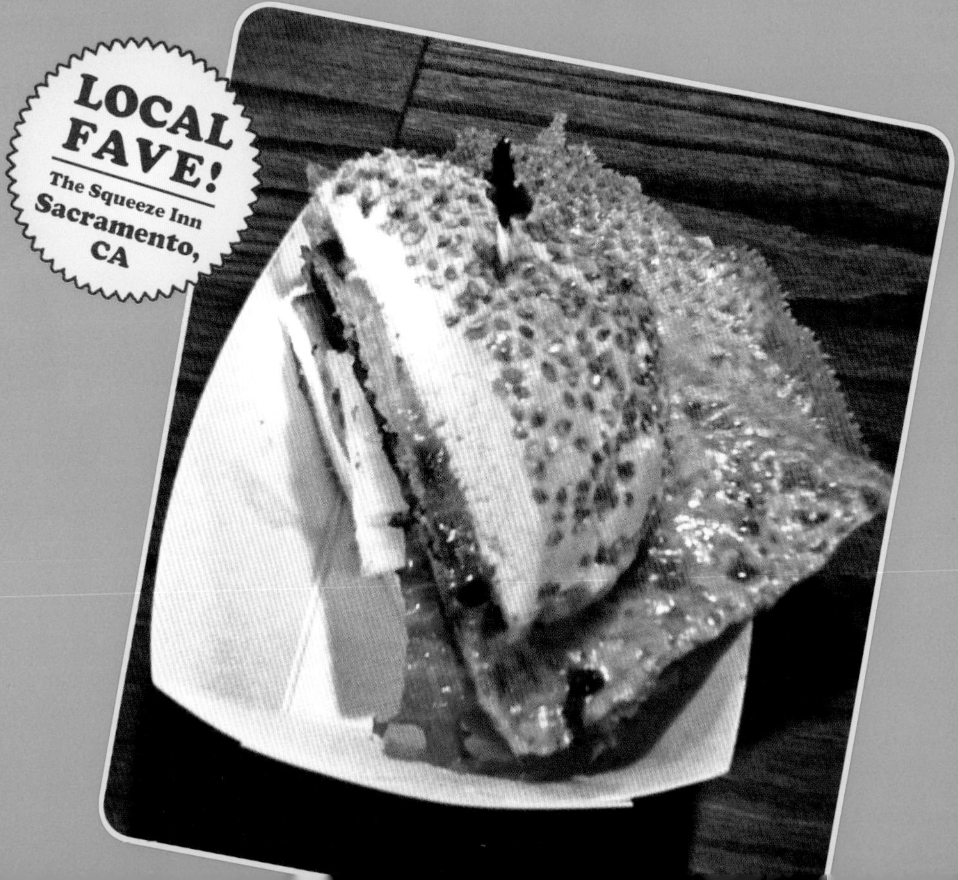

LOCAL FAVE!

The Squeeze Inn
Sacramento, CA

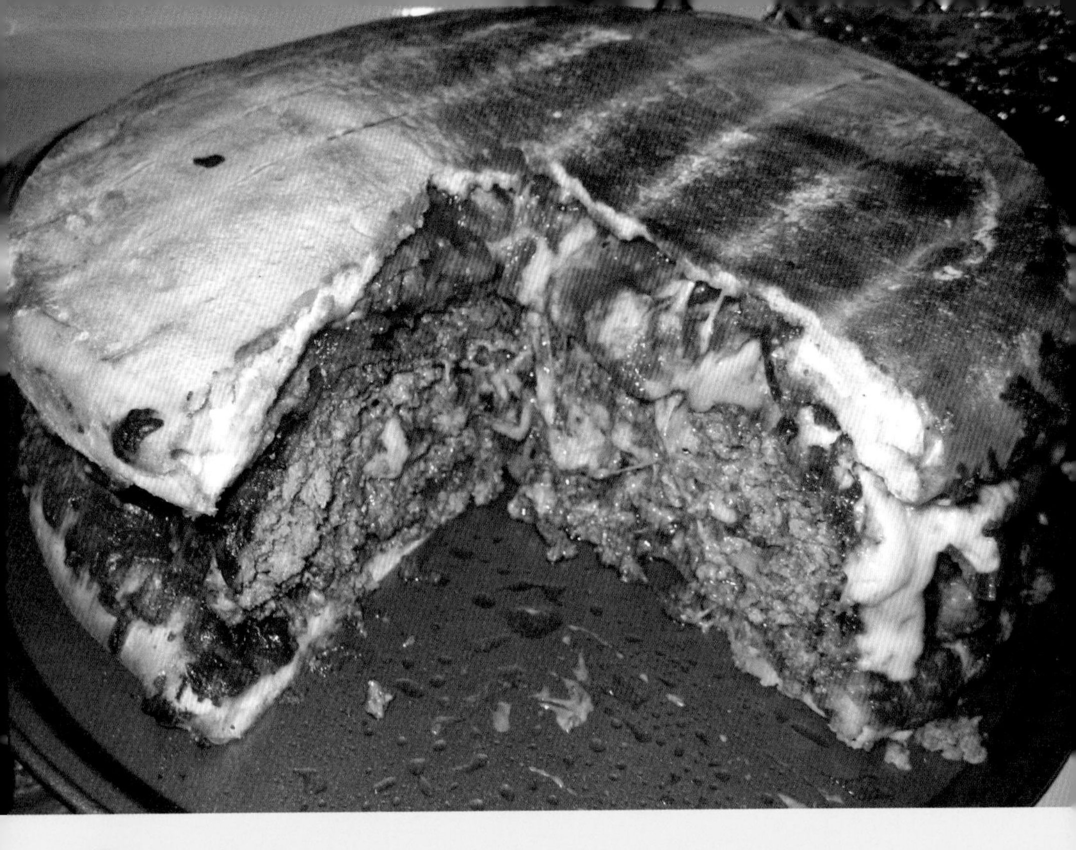

It was Super Bowl Sunday and I knew I had to conceive a meal that would truly dazzle the eyes and blow some gourds. To me, the Super Bowl is the one event of the year that capitalizes on everything that makes America awesome. Thus the choice was clear: create an awesome combination of three gloriously fat-filled American foods—bacon, pizza and hamburgers!

—DUSTIN SCHIRER (CREATOR OF THE BACON CHEESE PIZZA BURGER)

Bacon Cheese Pizza Burger

Recipe by Dustin Schirer

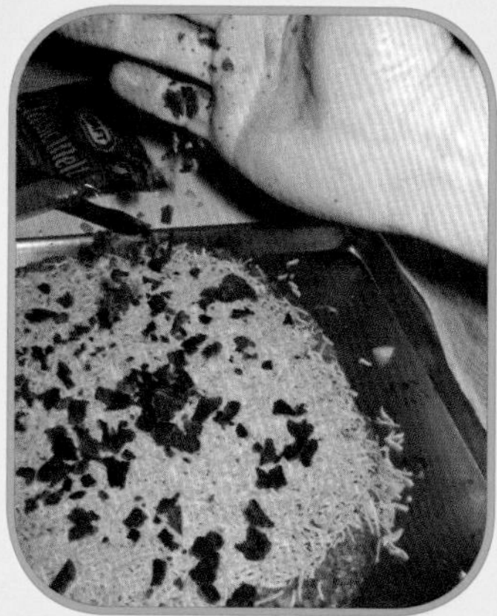

1–2 lbs bacon
3 lbs burger meat
6 eggs
Sliced pepper Jack cheese
Shredded Colby-Jack cheese
2 meat pizzas

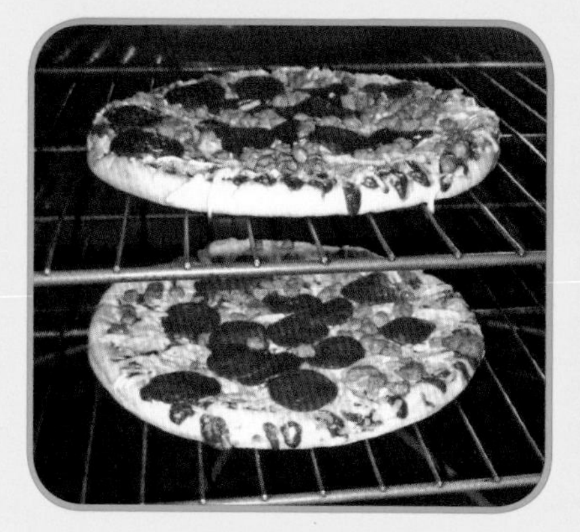

Fry bacon, then drain the grease and chop the bacon. Mix hamburger meat with eggs. Divide the meat mixture into two large patties. Cover one burger with shredded cheese, then top with chopped bacon. Place the second burger on top of the first; squish the burgers together. Sprinkle bacon on top in the shape of a dream catcher. Cook burger at 350° F for 1½ hours. Sprinkle with remaining bacon. Bake the pizzas in the oven. Remove pizzas and top with remaining shredded cheese. Transfer the burger onto one pizza. Top with the remaining pizza.

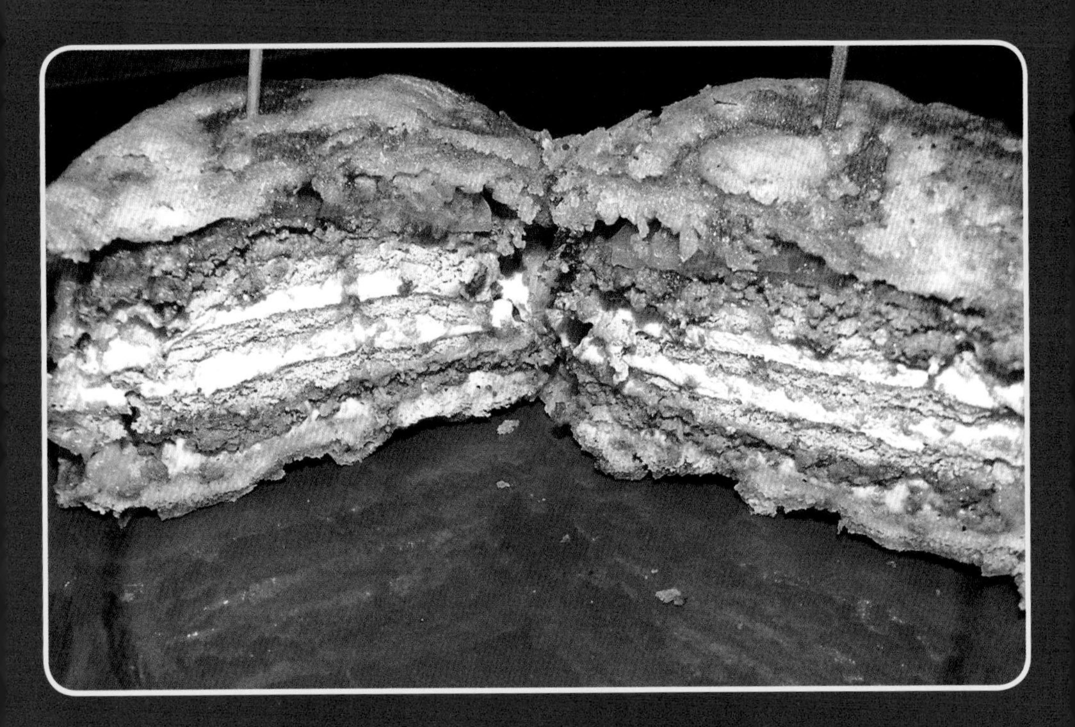

Deep-Fried MoonPie Burger

A MoonPie in between two McDonald's double cheeseburger patties, all deep-fried.

Fattie Melt

A bacon cheeseburger with grilled-cheese sandwiches as buns.

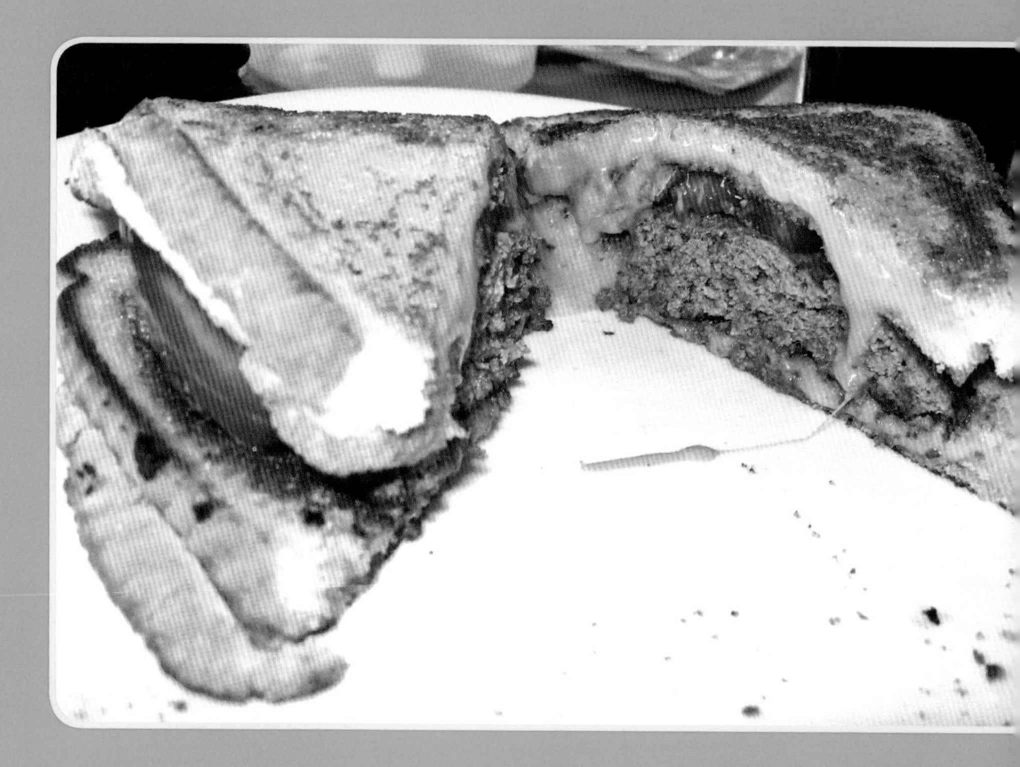

Mega Burger 2.0

Recipe by Billy

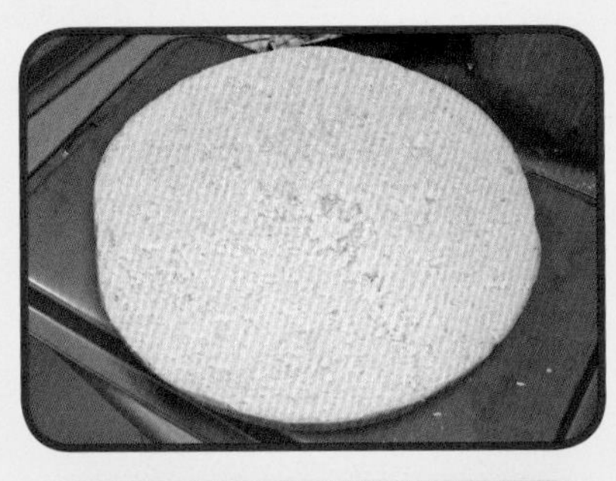

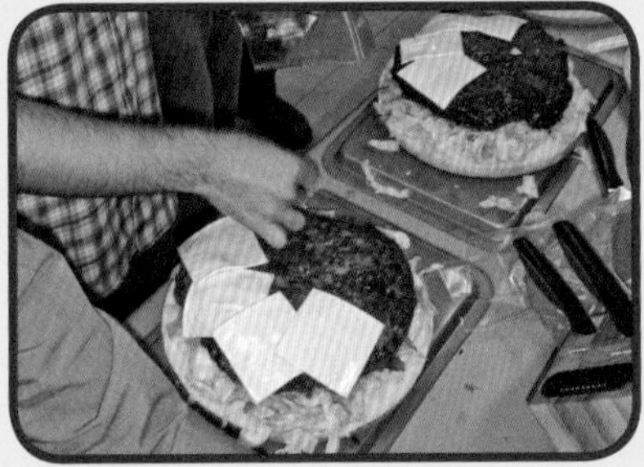

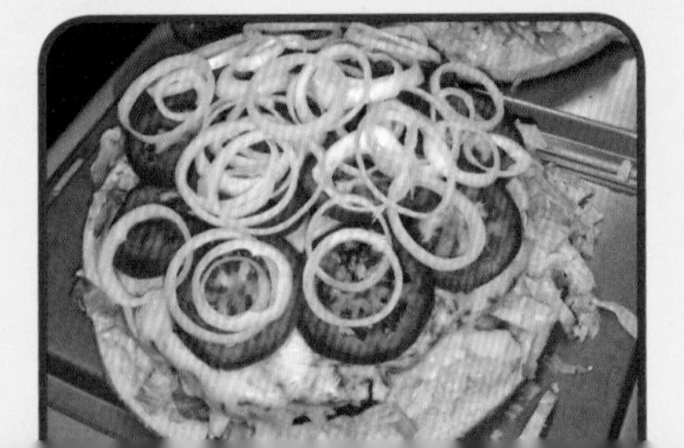

1 head iceberg lettuce
4 tomatoes
2 onions
1 white bread mix
2 ½ tbsp of water
24 slices cheese
1 sprinkle of sesame seeds
2 White Wings Hamburger Helper
1 cup ketchup
3/4 cup mayonnaise
1/2 cup mustard
5 eggs
25 oz dill pickles

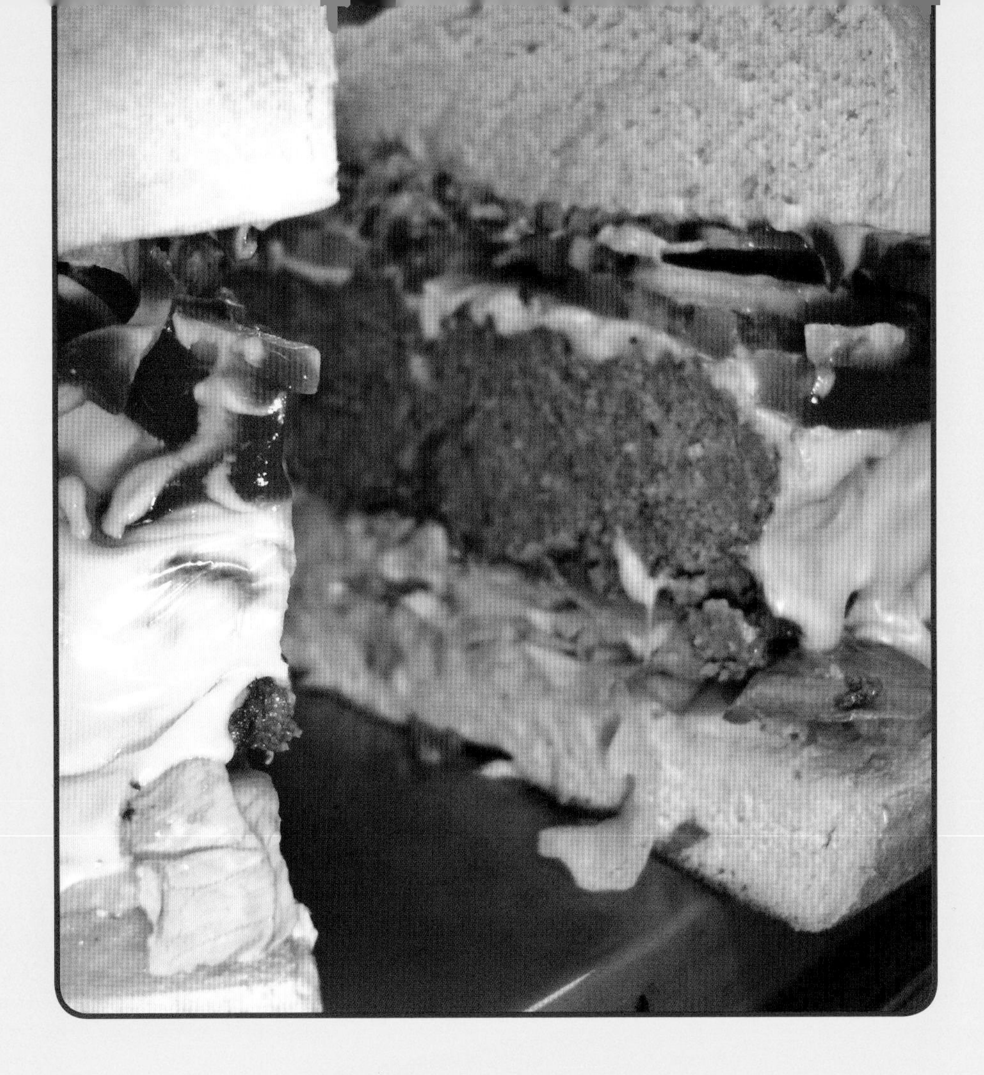

Quadruple Bypass Burger

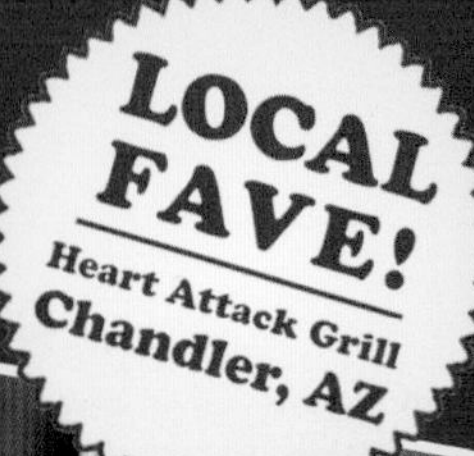

Acknowledgments

In no particular order . . .

Jessica would like to thank: my partner/roommate/boyfriend, Richard, for being a positive force in getting this site off the ground, creating killer design ideas and for knowing when to let his strong-willed (and usually right!) partner get her way.

I'd also like to thank our literary agent, Daniel Greenberg, and all of our contributors and fans who have made the site—and this book—everything it is.

A very special thanks goes to our intern and friend, Whitney Jefferson, for her endless help and loose interpretation of "regular work hours."

Thank you to Diana Levine for making us look hip and skinny.

Many thanks to David Karp and the Tumblr team for hosting our blog, and greeting our suggested account features/customizations with the same openness as our video-rap performances.

Thank you, Mom, for offering to buy "every copy" of this book. Thank you, Dad, for all your business and life advice, and thank you, Erik, for sending me regular IMs that say: "omg my sister's famous."

I'd also like to thank Mack Williams for his design input and Joe Garden for the hilarious Foreword.

Thank you to all my friends for their high fives, support, and general awesomeness during this process.

Last but not least, thanks to our publishing team, my patient editors at Urlesque.com, and of course, the Internet.

Richard would like to thank: my amazingly talented girlfriend, whose ability to see the larger picture and be the most detail-oriented person I know always amazes me, along with her scheduling abilities and her gift for juggling a million different things at once with Nazi-like precision. This entire project wouldn't have been a fraction of what it is without you, Jess.

My trusty video department companion Mike Byhoff for staying late while we were wrapped up in countless book-related meetings.

Our amazing intern, Whitney Jefferson.

Nick Denton for always gleefully supporting my often half-baked, and in this case deep-fried, side projects.

Will Leitch for thanking me in his book, *God Save the Fan,* which at some point I will get around to reading—promise!

The amateur food porn community—this book wouldn't exist without you.

All of our friends who kept our identities secret for so long.

Most of all, I would like to thank my mom and dad for raising me vegetarian. :)

Contributor Index

14-Pie Pie
Ben McLeod, Alex Chan, George Organ, Allan McGregor, John Psegianakis, Joel Roncevich, and Peter Schmidt

100x100 In-N-Out Burger
(Twitter) @whatupwilly

29,559 Calorie Sandwich
Josh Mattson

All-Day-Long Sandwich of Dreams
Rosa, Paul, Tara—Ensaladagranada.blogspot.com

The American Dream
Nick Amosson

BA-K-47
Nicholas Hamon—thisisfreakingridiculous.com

Bacon Apple Pie
Recipe: Phoebe Owens and Michael Crozier
Photo: Scott Kveton

Bacon Beeritos
Edward Shen and Michael Ybarra, sheniferous (Flickr)

Bacon Burger Dog
Recipe: Texas Burger Guy
Photo: Mark Guppy

Bacon Cake
Jenny Gant and Jennifer Wong

Bacon Cheese Pizza Burger
Photo and copy: Dustin Schirer

Bacon Chocolate Chip Cookies
Maggie Fritz-Morkin

Bacon Cinnamon Rolls
Andy Phelan

The Bacone
Recipe: Christian Williams and Melissa Tillman
Copy: Christian Williams
Photo: Scott Kveton

Bacon Explosion Wellington
Thomas Trumble (TPapi on Flickr)
Rob Morton—BaconJew.com

Bacon Mac and Cheese Meatloaf
Kyle Kestell and Jameel Winter—VIVAHATE.com

Bacon Weave Cheese Roll-up
Eric Rosendahl and Daniel Cooper, Esq. (Flickr)

The Beer Barrel Belly Buster
Jvc_scout_mom (Flickr)

Beth's 12-Egg Omelette
gizmo2z (Flickr)

Breakfast Fatty
Recipe: Thomas Lester
Photo: Robert Kemper and everyone at TheSmokeRing.com forums

Burrito Cake
Cary and Jeremy Hammond

Cadbury Egg Nog
Seth Porges

Candy Sushi
Kim Becker—mommyknows.com

Carnegie Deli Reuben
Ryan

Cheesy French Toast
Helenebear

Chocolate-Covered Bacon
Bill Lambert, Erickson Design

Corn Dog Pizza
Jason Eliaser

The Cornhole
Joe T. and EOB

Country Breakfast Parfait
Marah Anderson and Gus Straub

Country Pancake Wrap
Lawrence Weibman—NYCFoodGuy.com

Cracklin'
Kristen Zeiber

The Deep-Fried Brownie Ball
Sarah Hopp

Deep-Fried Cadbury Crème Egg
Kerryn Findlay

Deep-Fried Coke
Stephen Witherden

Deep-Fried Deviled Egg
Stephanie Bunn, Dispensing Happiness

Deep-Fried Grilled-Cheese Sandwich
Ben Chan (bent0box on Flickr)

Deep-Fried Mars Bar
Christian Cable

Deep-Fried MoonPie
Brian Gregory—cheapblueguitar.com

Deep-Fried MoonPie Burger
Zach Zanassi, Jonathan Iwazaki, Natalie Marrs, Alex Cornelison and Tyler Fitzgerald

Deep-Fried Oreo
Douglas Cheung

Deep-Fried Pop-Tart
melmyfinger (Flickr)

Deep-Fried S'more on a Stick
(Twitter) @emfred

Deep-Fried Twinkie
melmyfinger (Flickr)

Ditch Dogs
Greg Johnson—oatmealcookieguy.com

Donut Cake
Sarah Lyon (Hvyilnr on Flickr)

Elvis Donut
Keith and Corie Rein

Fattie Melt
Bill Binns

The Fat Tuesday
Bryan S. Thompson

Fried Guac Bites
Recipe: Rick Blakeley
Photo: Adam Pava—GuacBowl.com
Made by: Craig Anderson

Frito Pie
Recipe: Mona Meline
Photo: Jennifer Whalen (Flickr)

Garbage Plate
Dan Dangler

The G.B.M.F.
Ann

Gluttonator
Recipe: Chris Green and Olivia Osborne
Photo: Nicola Bowerbank

Gravy Pizza
Alexa Clark (Lex on Flickr)

Grilled Cheesecake Sandwich
Jessie—Cakespy.com

Hamburger Cake
Lisa Brockmeier

Hamdog
Noel Kersh—texasburgerguy.com

Happy Meal Pizza
myspace.com/djfirth

Heart Attack Sandwich
Lennon Day-Reynolds

Hot Beef Sundae
Tom Coates—plasticbag.org

Hot Dog Cake
Leslie Behrens

Hot Dog Crêpes
ZeBieler (Flickr)

The Kannibal
Lorraine Elliott—notquitenigella.com

Kenny & Zuke's DDD Reuben
Nick Zukin

Krispy Kreme Milk Shake
Recipe: Julia Schweizer
Photo: Lara Goetzl

Loco Moco
James Rubio—www.bigislandgrinds.com

Lucy Juicy
Wendy Eischen

Luther Burger
John McBomb (McBomb on Flickr)

Massive BLT
OlderBoy

McGangBang
Li-Han Lin (polaroid_factory on Flickr)—polaroid-factory.blogspot.com/

McNuggetini
Recipe: Georgia Hardstark and Alie Ward
Photo: Leah Hardstark

Meatabulous quote
Joel Richards

Meat Cake
Julia Brylinski for pongalong.com

Meat House
Joel Richards, Bo Zhang, and Alex Tse—easyjo.com

Meat Salad
Kyle and Ellen Gowen

Meat Ship
Joel Richards, Bo Zhang, and Alex Tse—easyjo.com

The Meatza
Victoria Wren

Mega Burger 2.0
Billy—Supersizedmeals.com

Monster Box
Baud Attitude

Monster Sandwich Pie
Stephen Dietz

Party Sandwick Cake
Melissa Cabral and Paul Copeland—super-junk.com

Peanut Butter Bacon Burger
Casey Bisson—MaisonBisson.com

Pizza Cone
Superlocal (Flickr)

The Pizza Hut Double Roll Pizza
Michael B.

Porkgasm
Catherine Schon and Zach Spier

Poutine
Recipe: Peter Dutton (Joe Shlabotnik on Flickr)
Copy: Rachel Sklar

Quadruple Bypass Burger
Clarence F. Jacobs

The Reggie Deluxe
Kamala Dolphin-Kingsley (Flickr)

Sandwich of Knowledge
Luke Berryman

Scotch Egg
Nic McPhee

Shake Shack Double Stack
FourteenSixty (Flickr)

Slim Jim Shooters
Alayne W.

The Slinger
Miss Weeza (Flickr)

Snack Stadium
Nate and Dave—BSBrewing.com

The Squeeze with Cheese
August

Taco Cake
Kiara Ramirez

Taco Town Taco
Doyle Dodd and Drew Sloan

TriMacta
jennifer.hasegawa (Flickr)

Tubby Dog
Andree Lau—ugonnaeatthat.com

Turducken
Adam Selwood—smoiled.com/adamselwood

Turkey Cake
zcakes07 (Flickr)

Twinkie Weiner Sandwich
Photo: Jessica Amason

White Castle Casserole
Mr. Dave—ridiculousfoodsociety.com

White Trash Burrito
Kyle Nabilcy

World's Largest Cheeto
Adam Frucci

About the Authors

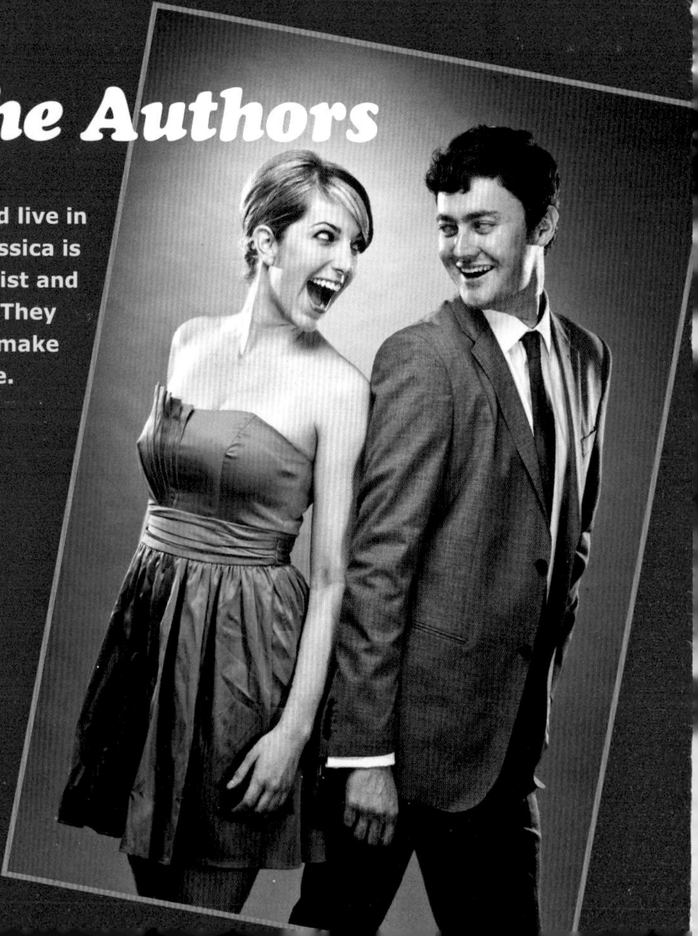

Jessica and Richard live in New York City. Jessica is a blogger/journalist and Richard is a video editor. They throw media parties and make trouble wherever possible.